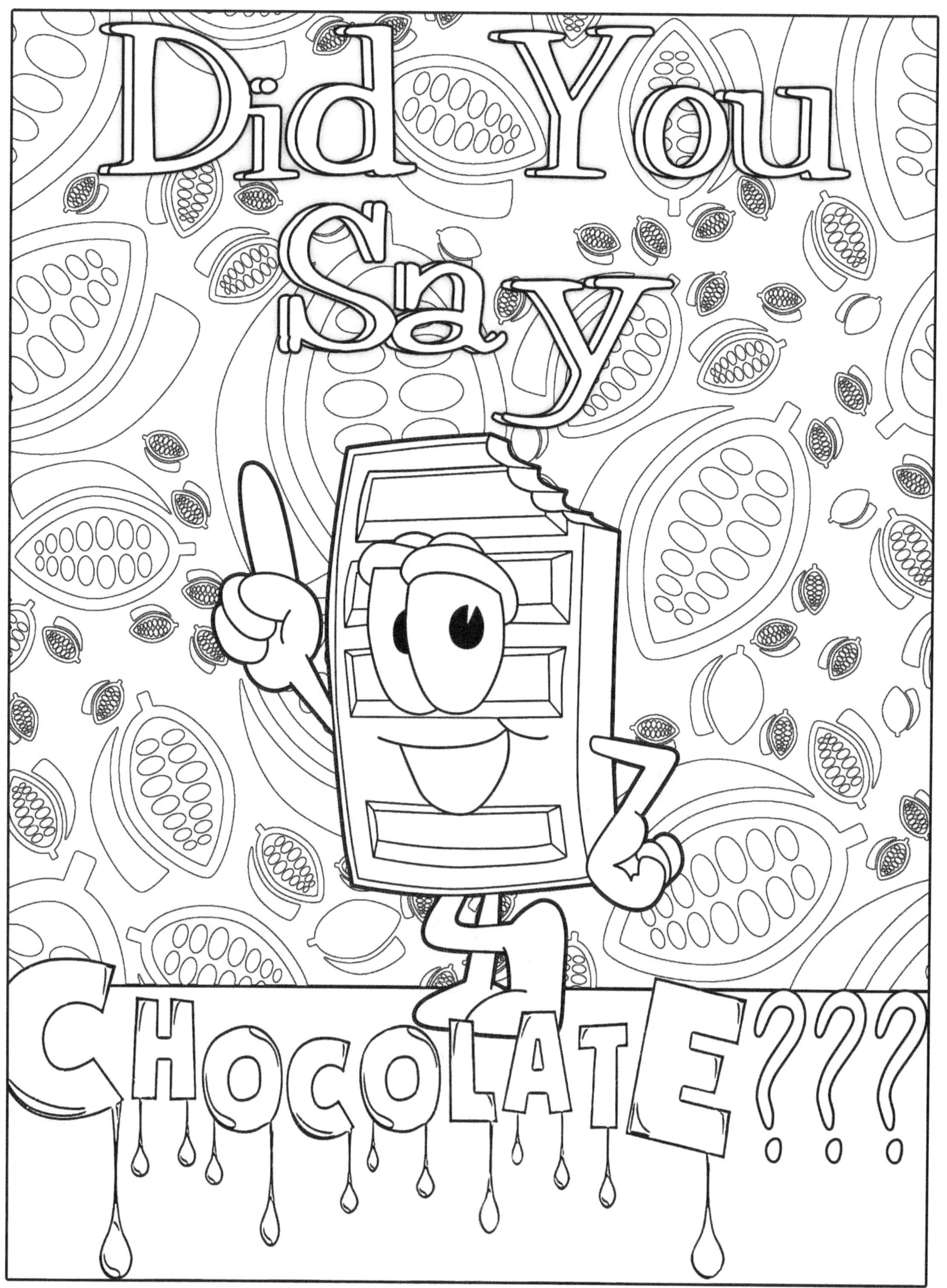

Did You
Say
Chocolate???

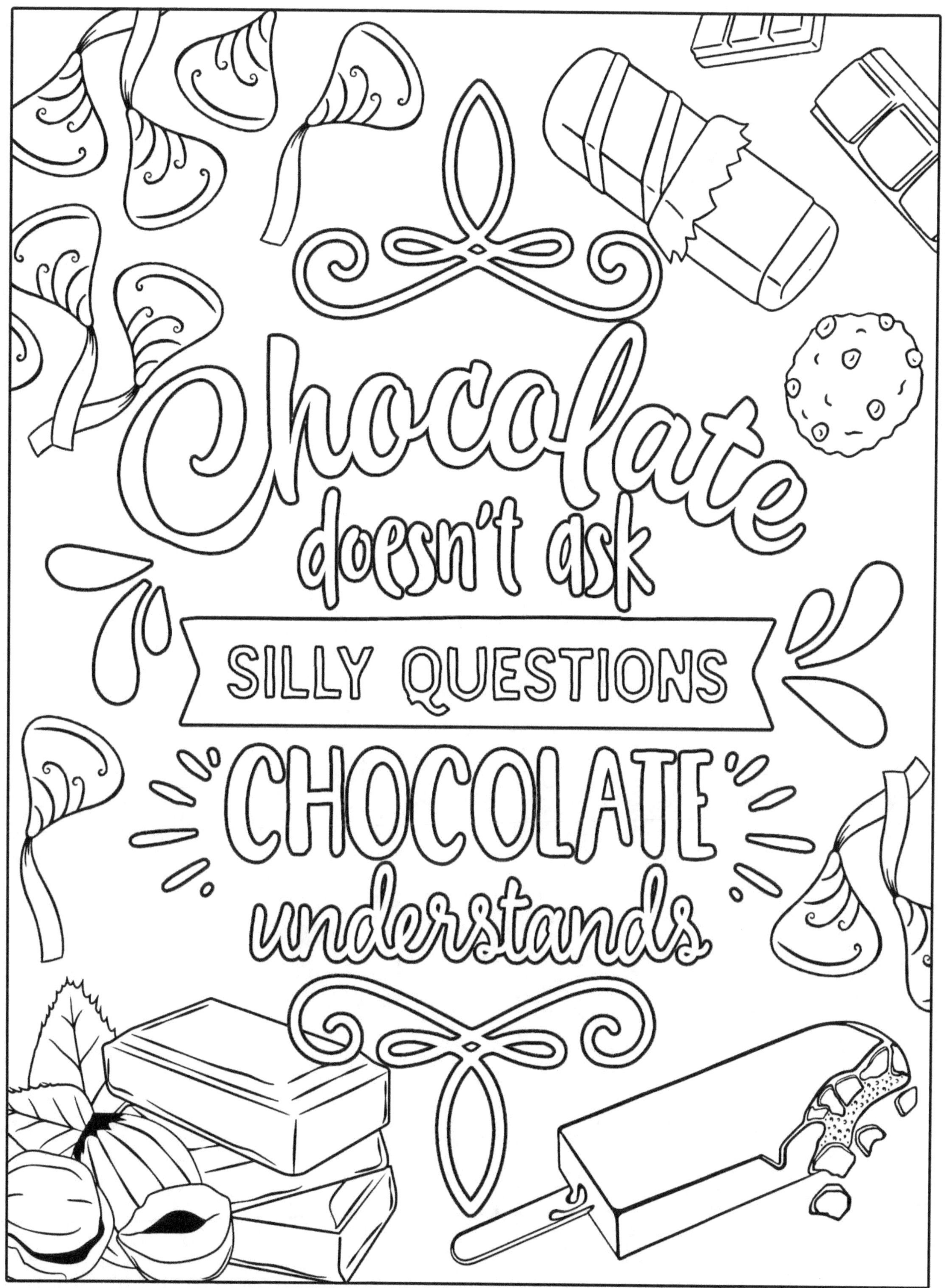

Chocolate
doesn't ask
SILLY QUESTIONS
"CHOCOLATE"
understands

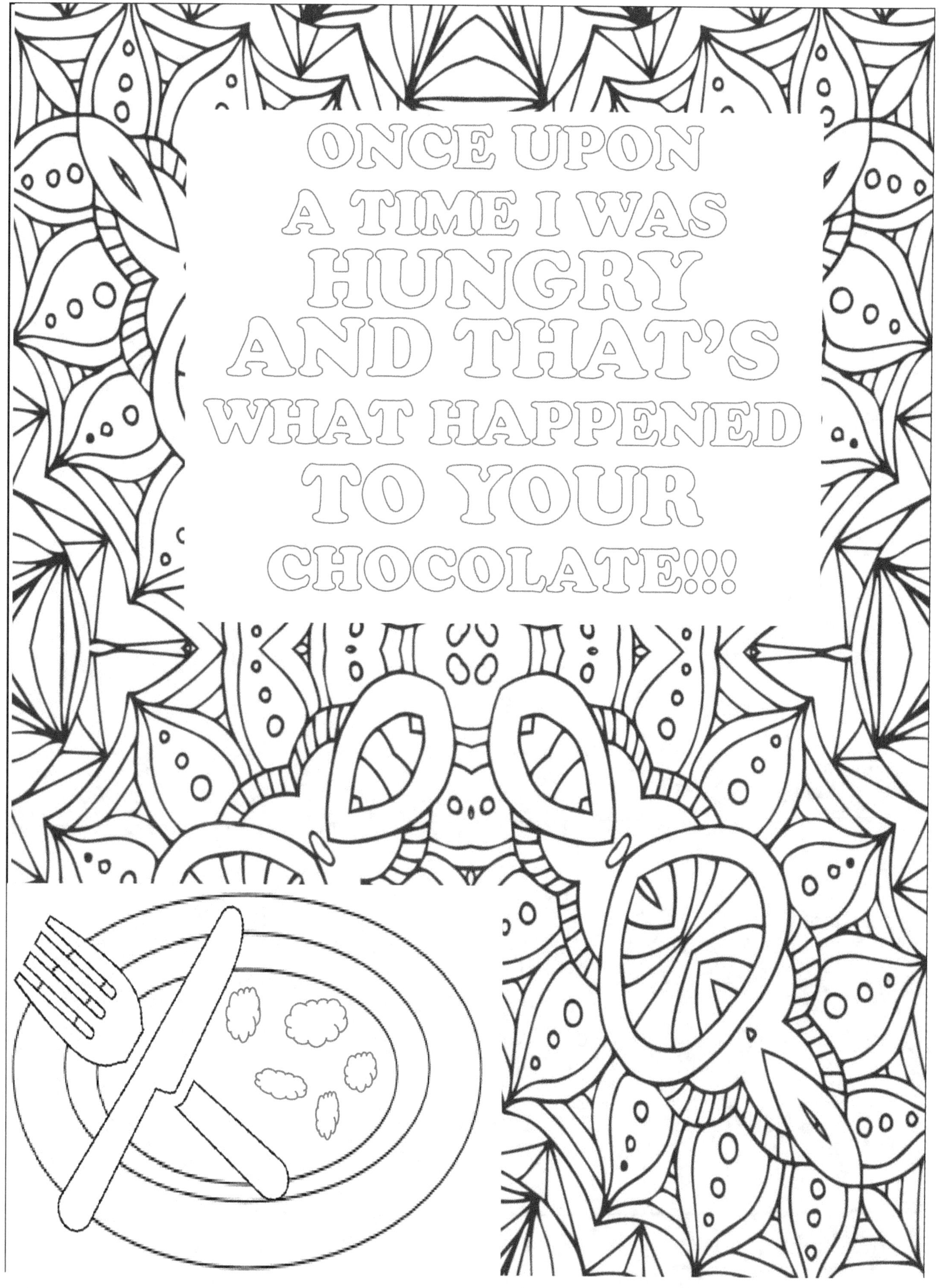

ONCE UPON
A TIME I WAS
HUNGRY
AND THAT'S
WHAT HAPPENED
TO YOUR
CHOCOLATE!!!

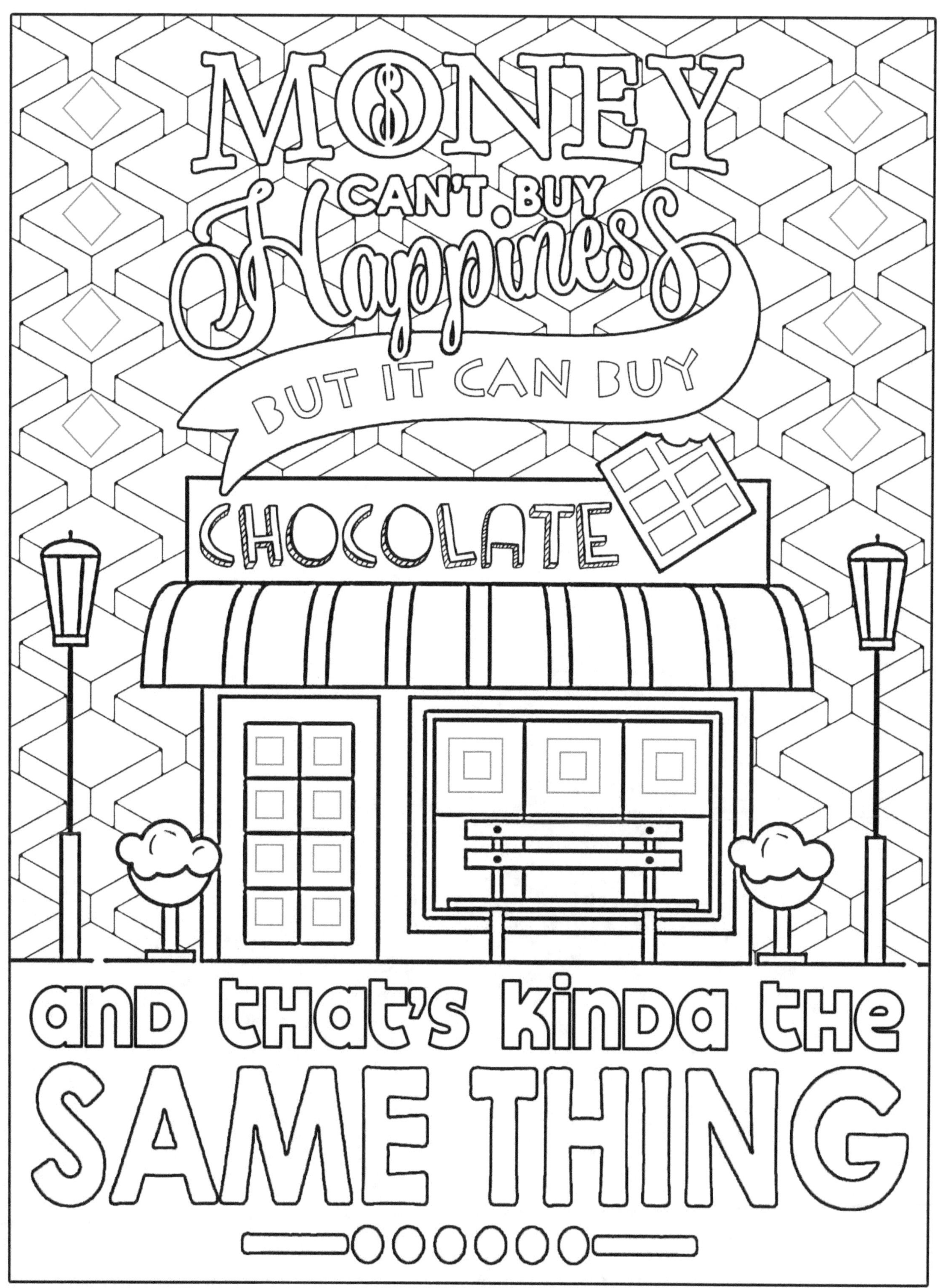

MONEY
CAN'T BUY
Happiness
BUT IT CAN BUY
CHOCOLATE
and that's kinda the
SAME THING

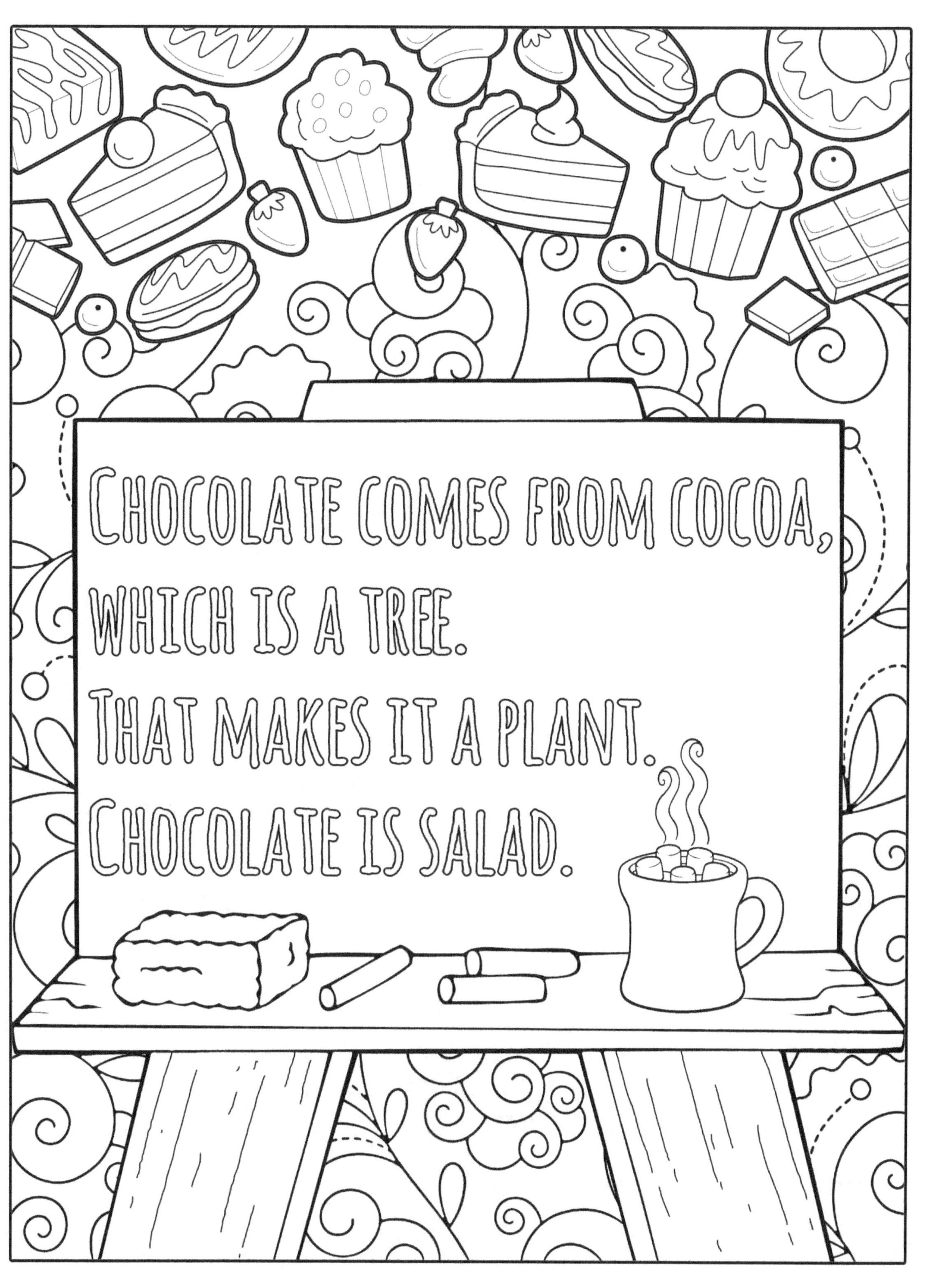

Chocolate comes from cocoa,
which is a tree.
That makes it a plant.
Chocolate is salad.

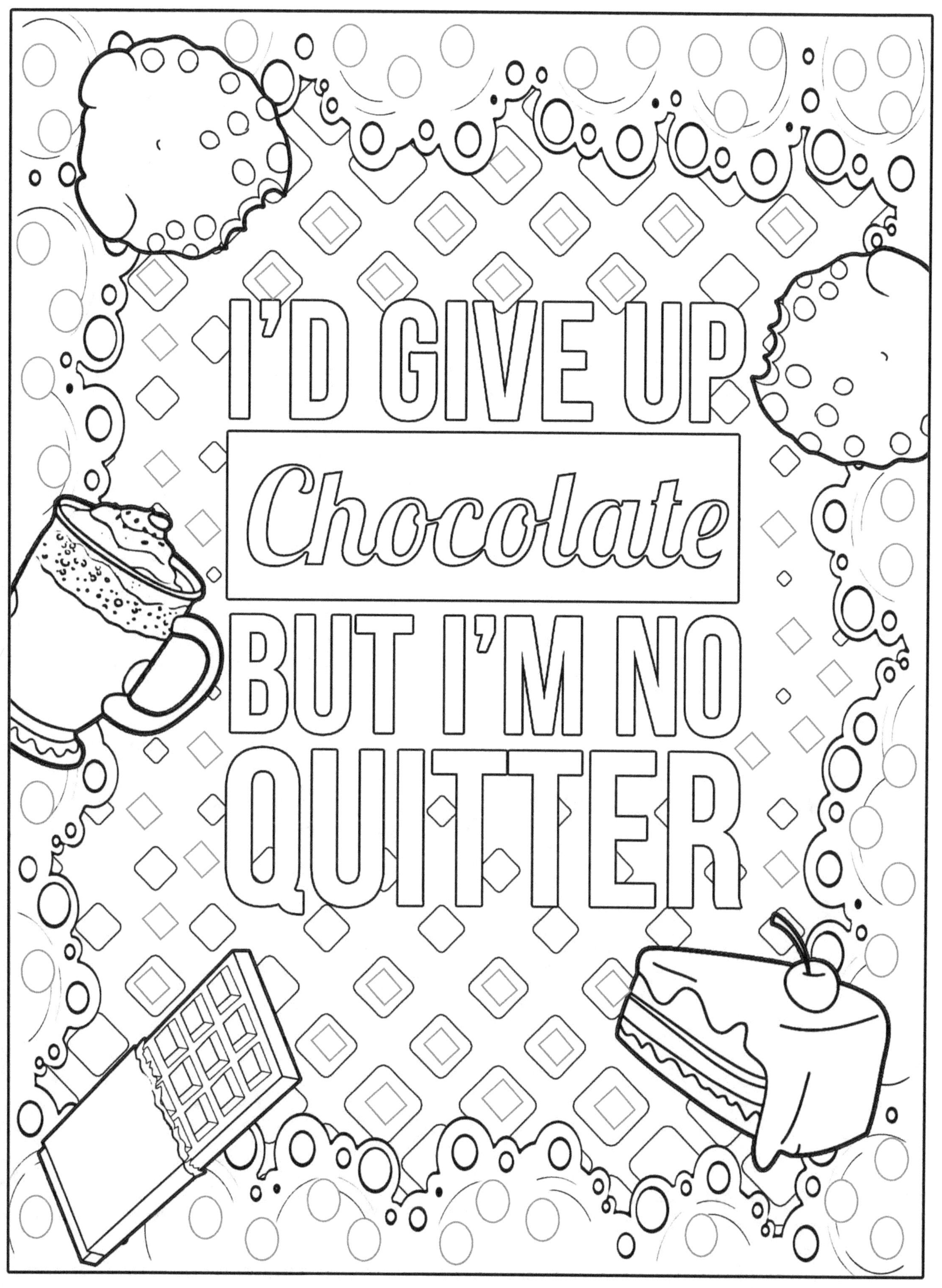

I'D GIVE UP
Chocolate
BUT I'M NO
QUITTER

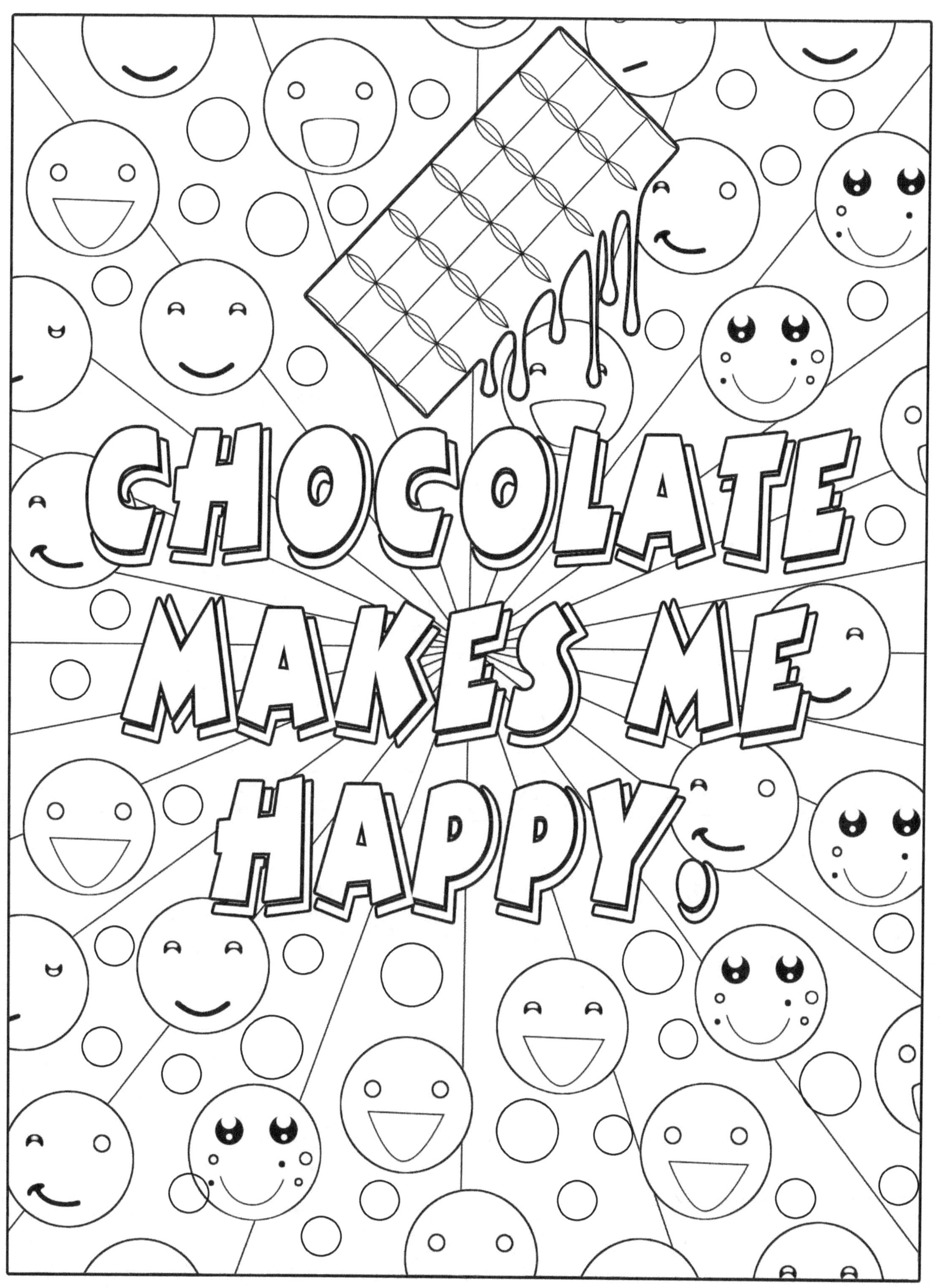

CHOCOLATE MAKES ME HAPPY.

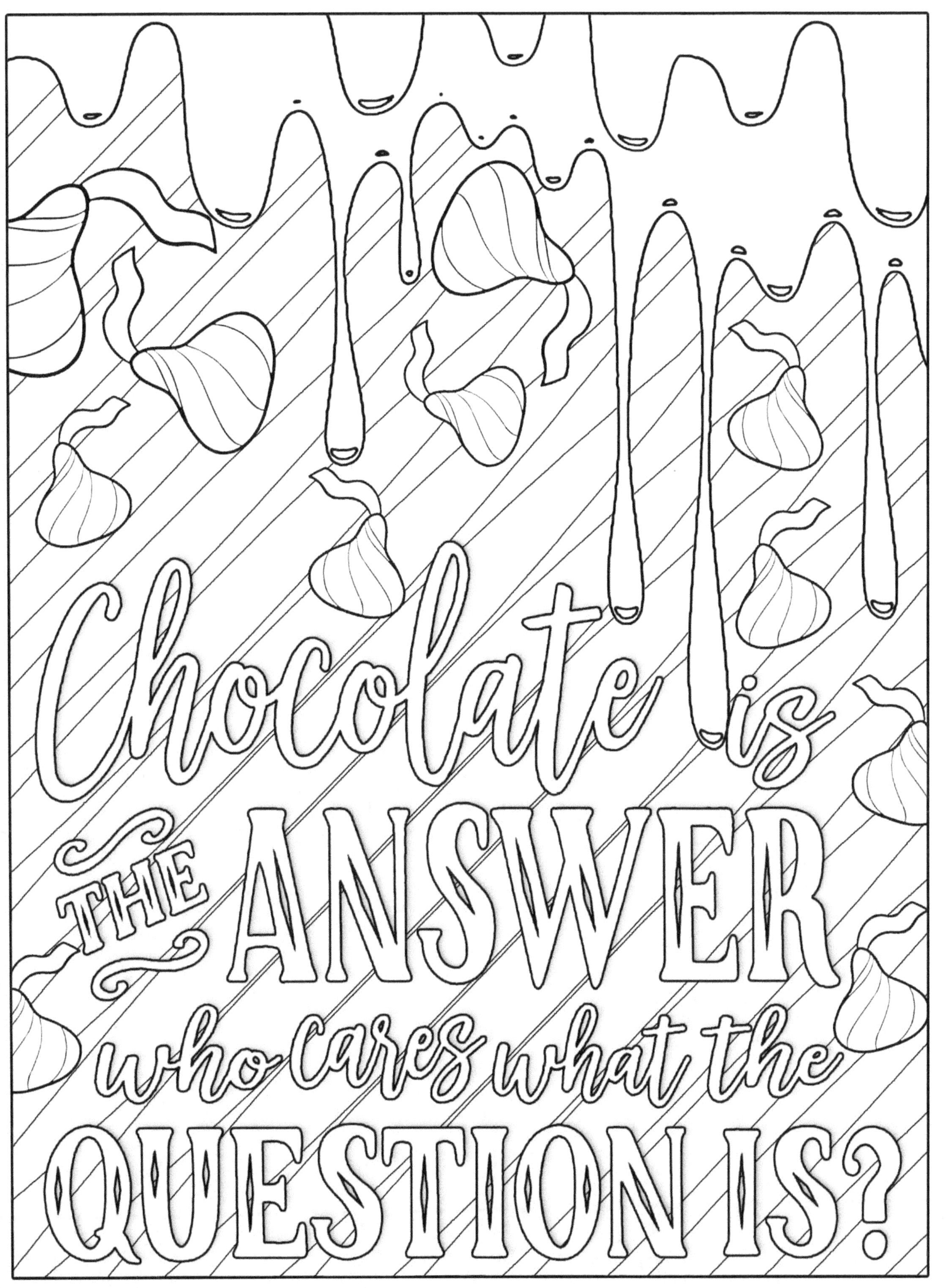

Chocolate is
the ANSWER
who cares what the
QUESTION IS?

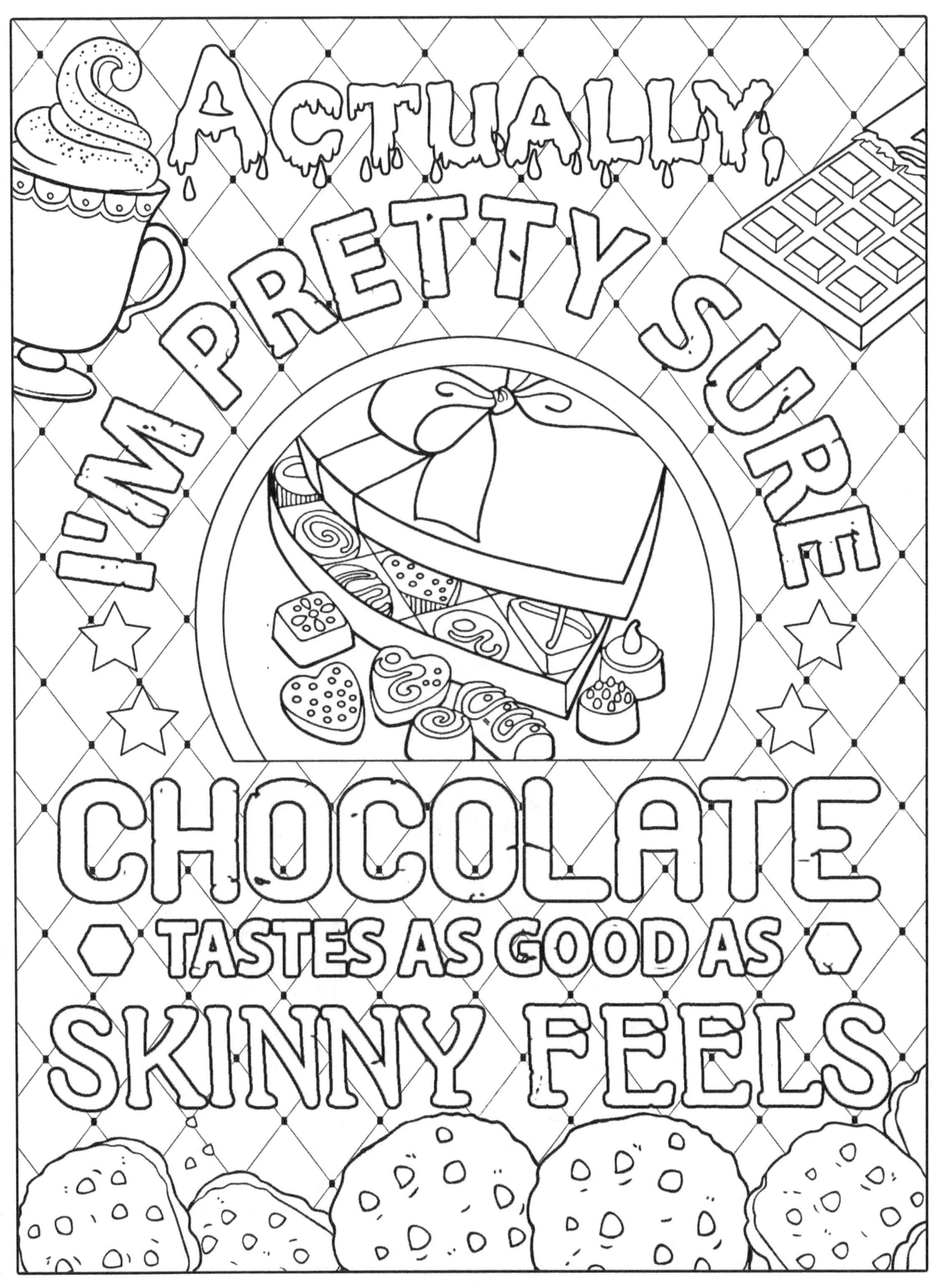

'SACTUALLY,
I'M PRETTY SURE
CHOCOLATE
TASTES AS GOOD AS
SKINNY FEELS

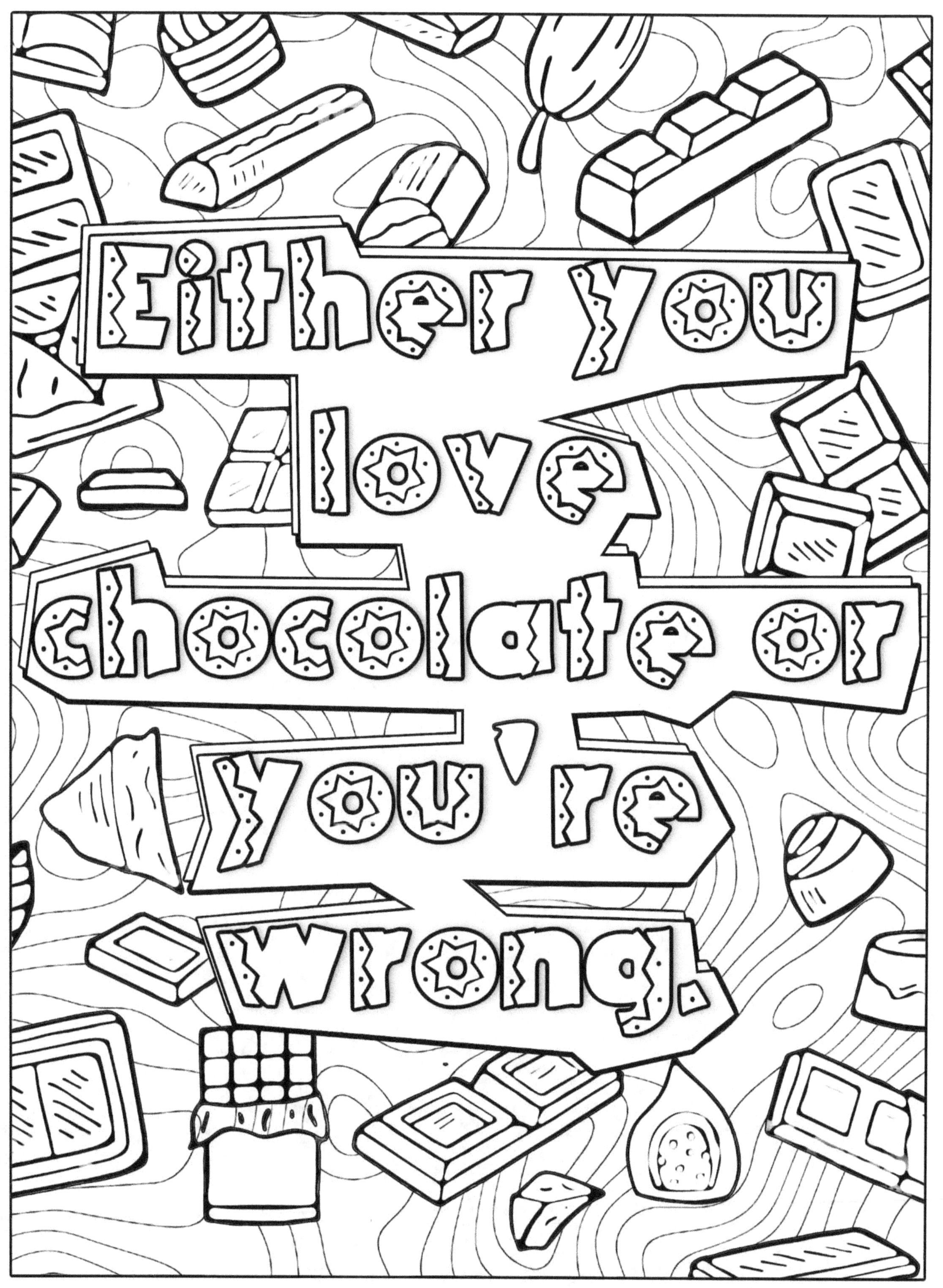

Either you
love
chocolate or
you're
wrong.

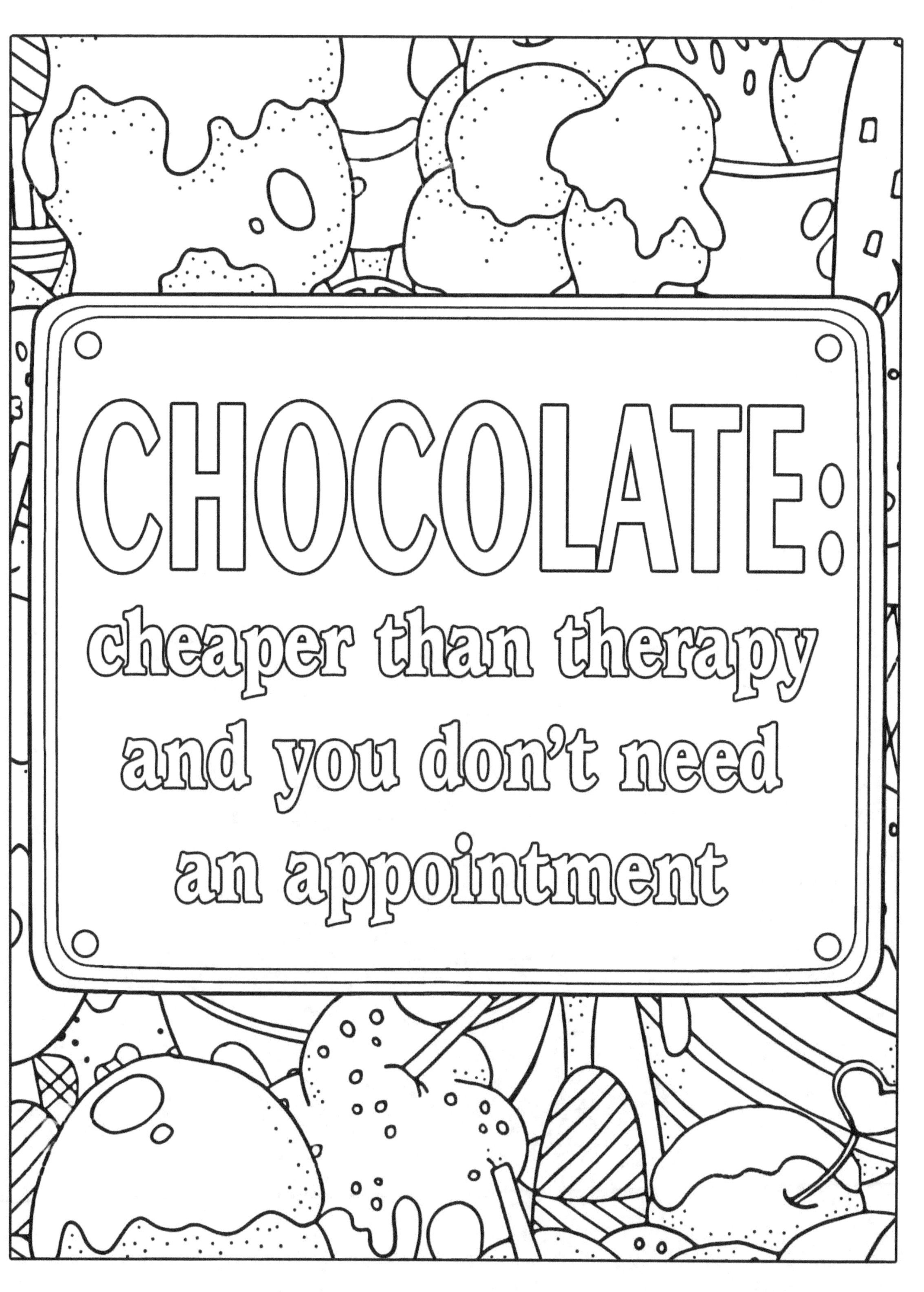

CHOCOLATE:
cheaper than therapy
and you don't need
an appointment

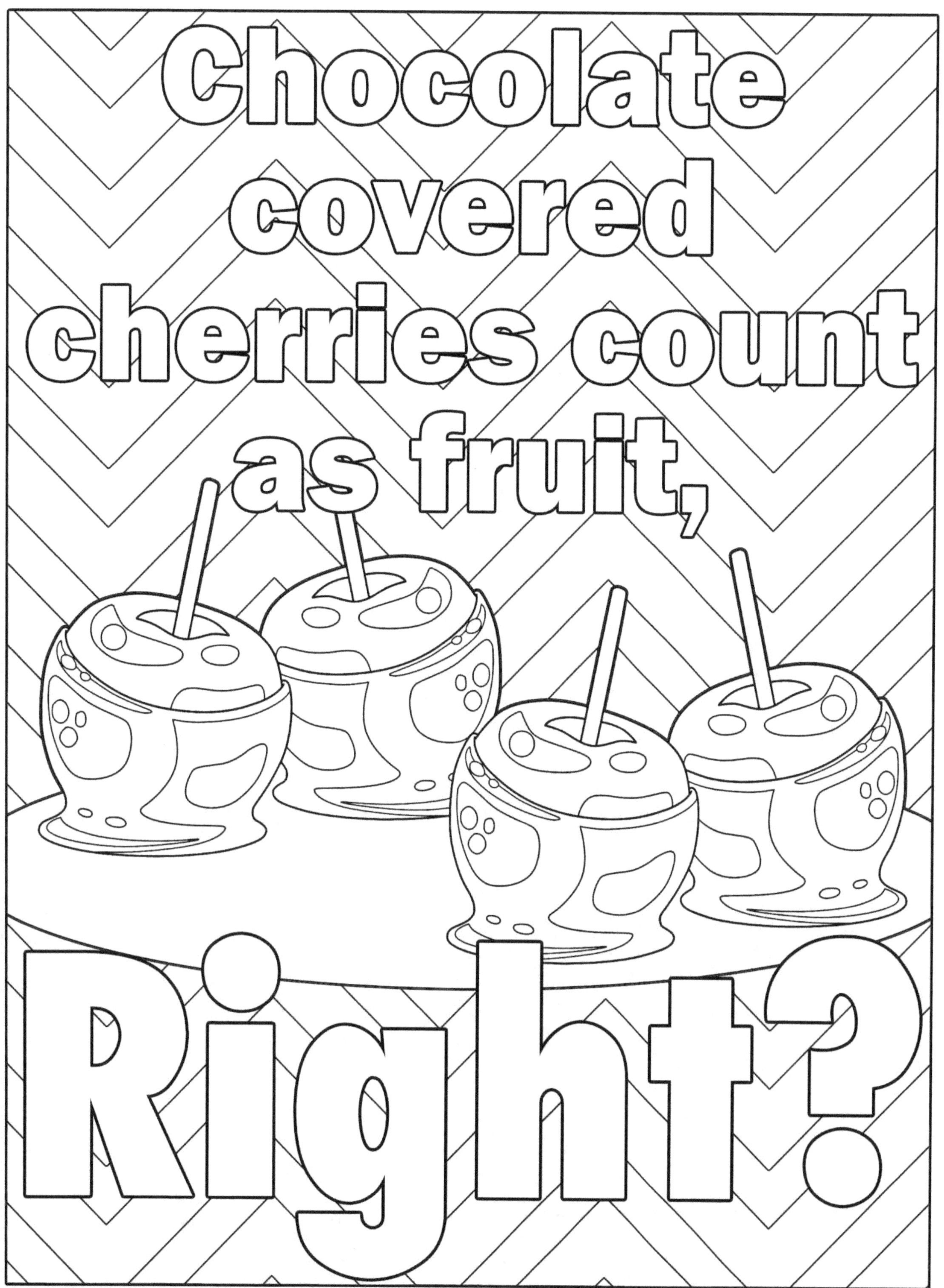

Chocolate covered cherries count as fruit,
Right?

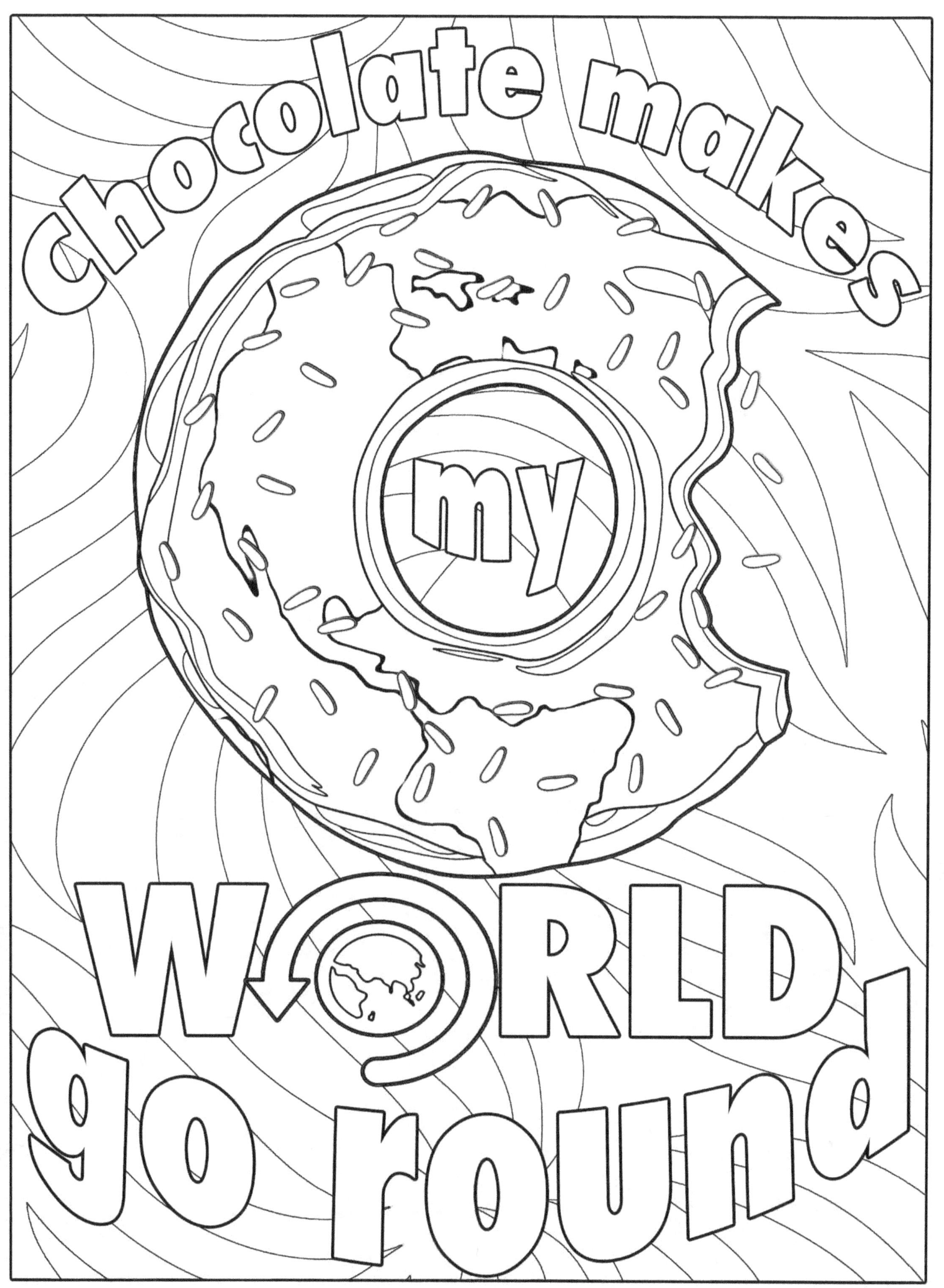

chocolate makes
my
WORLD
go round

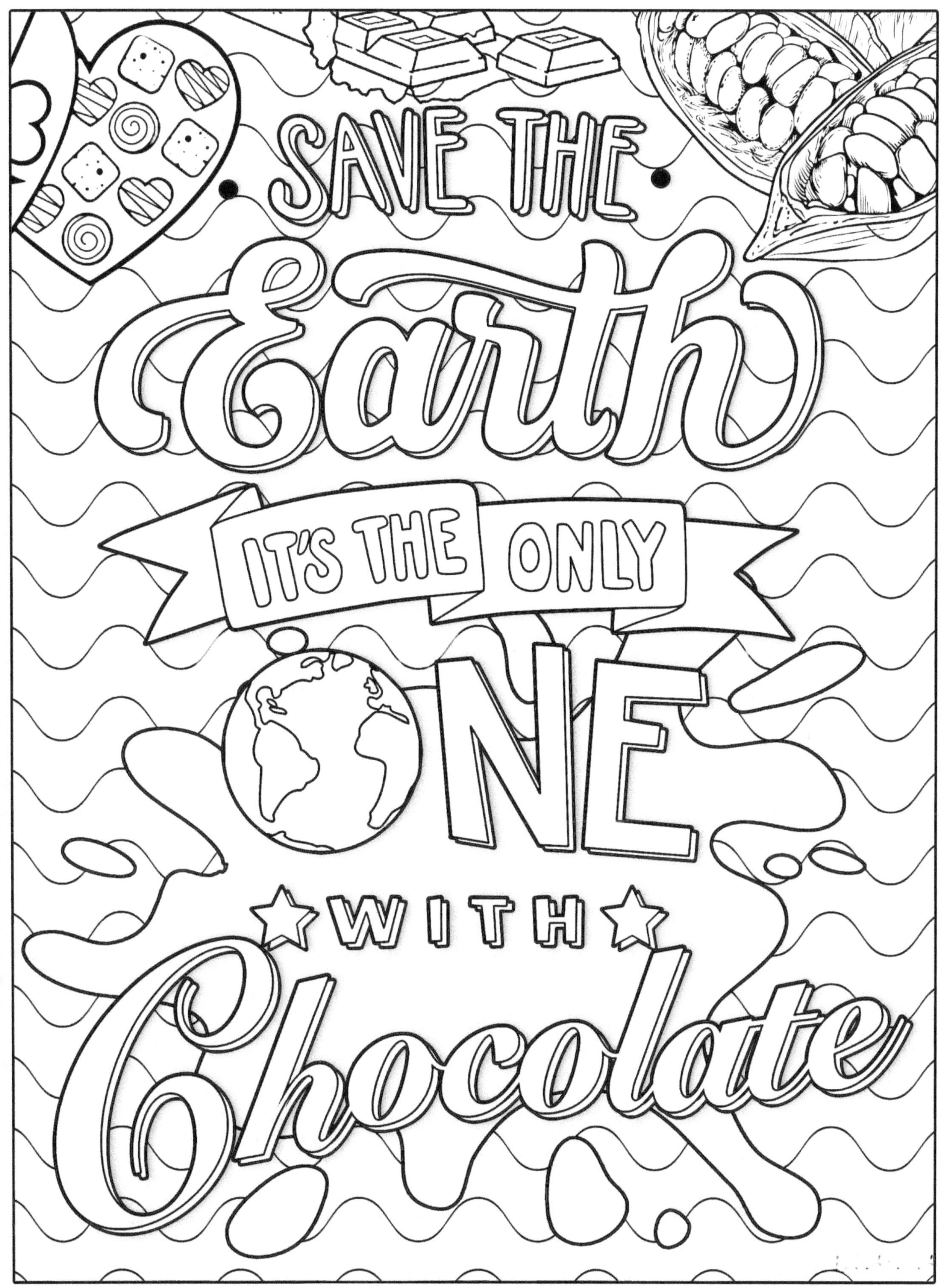

SAVE THE
Earth
IT'S THE ONLY
ONE
WITH
Chocolate

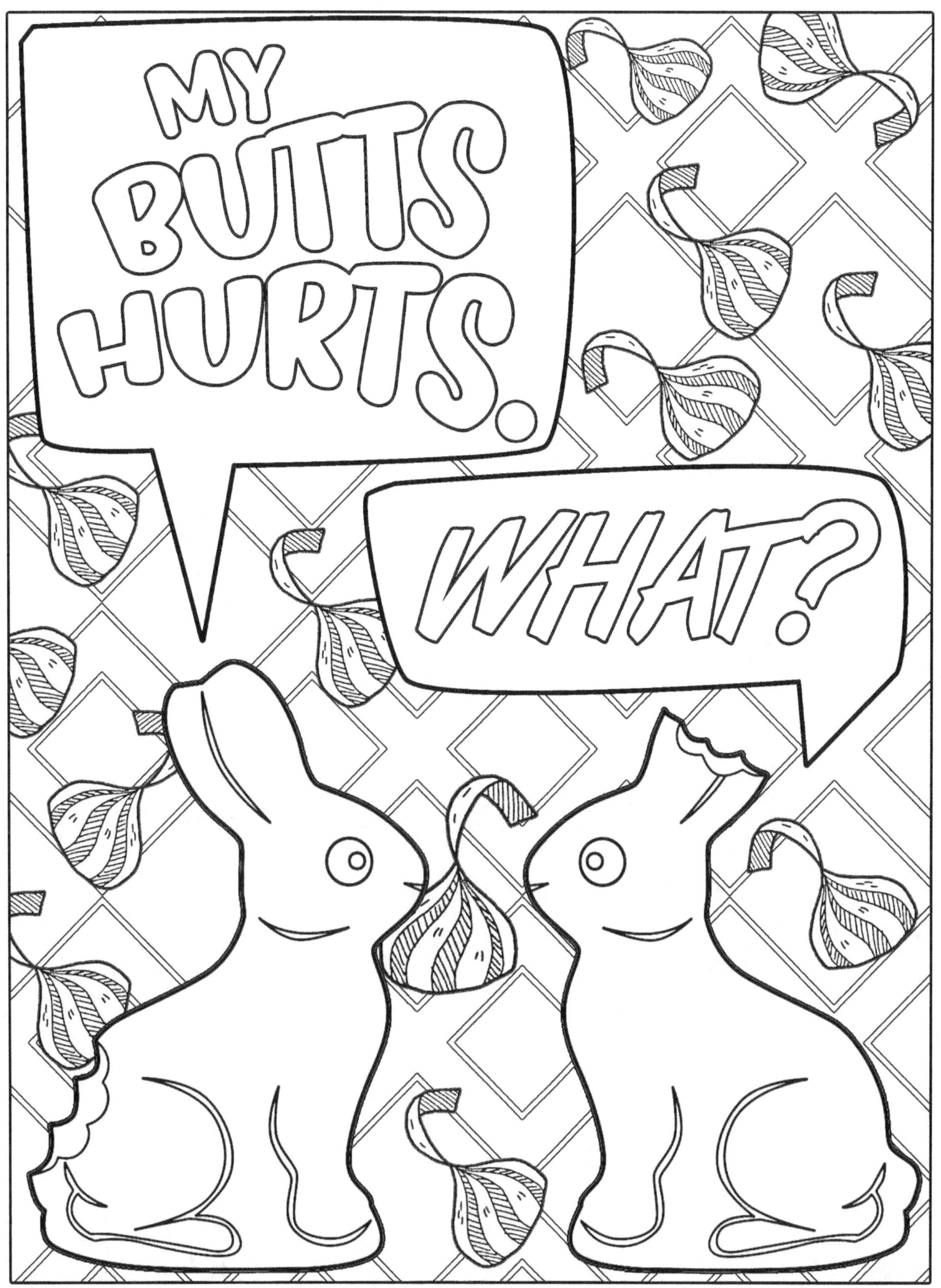

MY BUTTS HURTS.
WHAT?

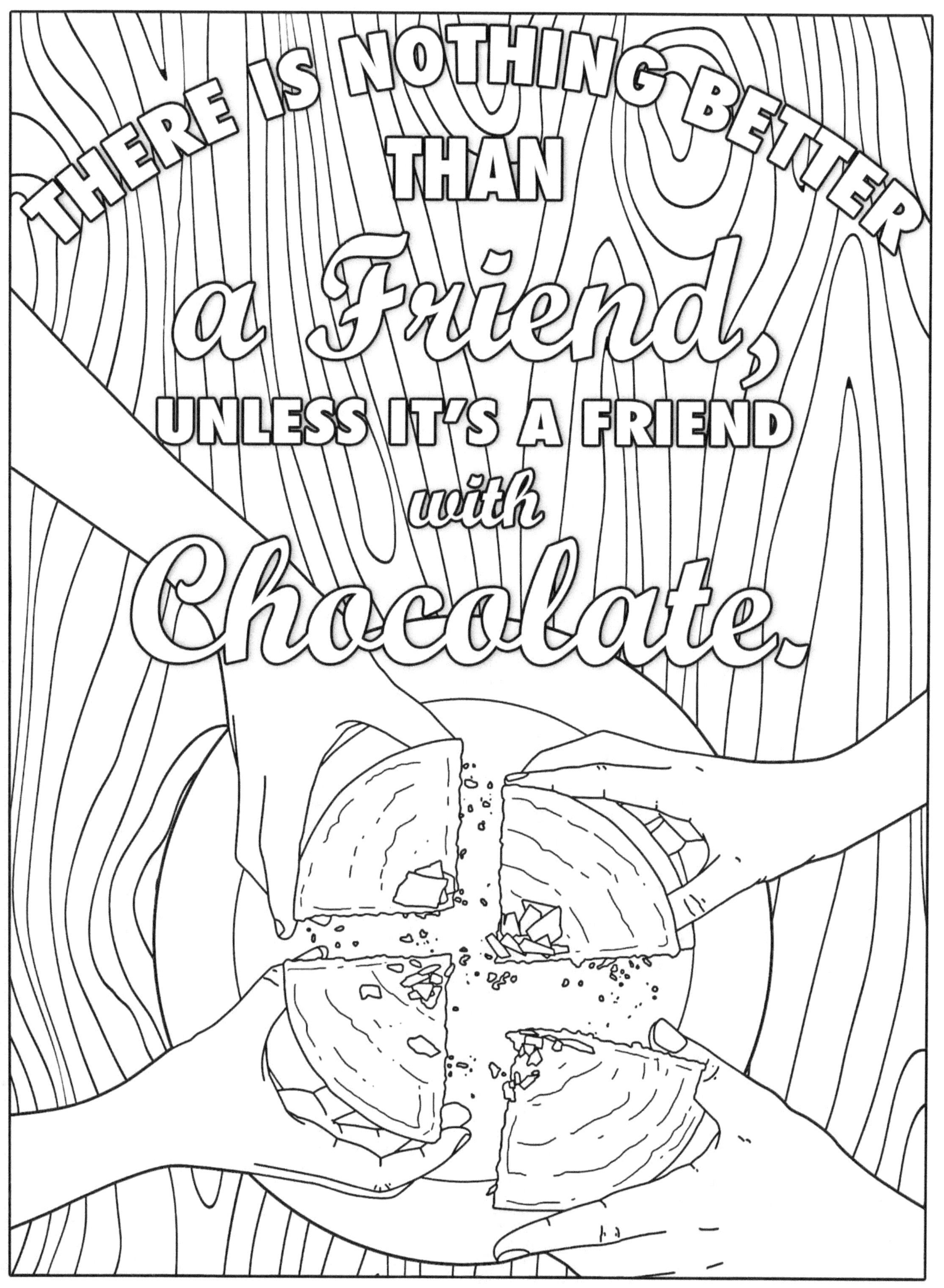

THERE IS NOTHING BETTER
THAN
a Friend,
UNLESS IT'S A FRIEND
with
Chocolate.

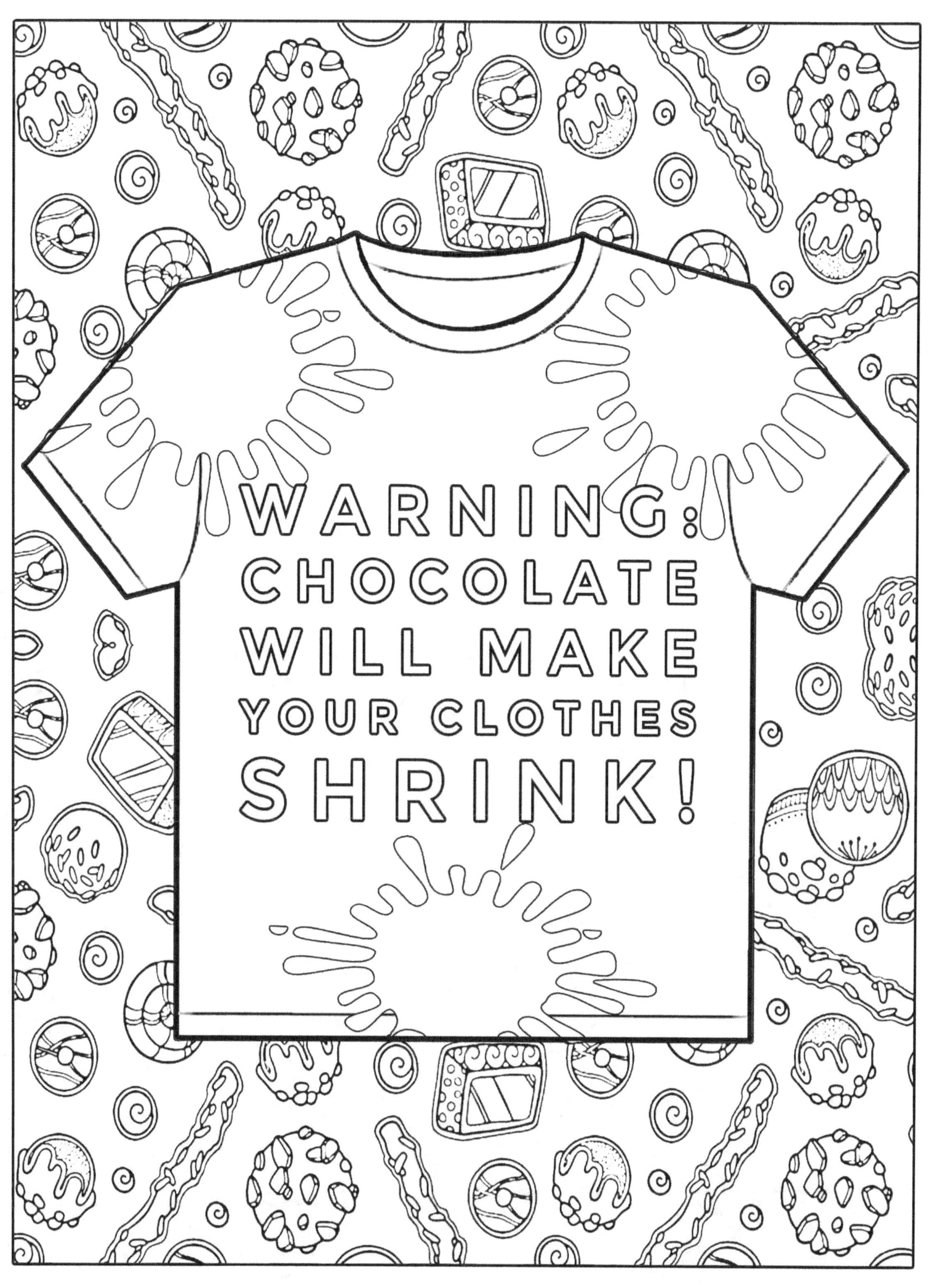

WARNING:
CHOCOLATE
WILL MAKE
YOUR CLOTHES
SHRINK!

ADMIST ALL THE CHAOS THERE IS...

Chocolate and Ice Cream!

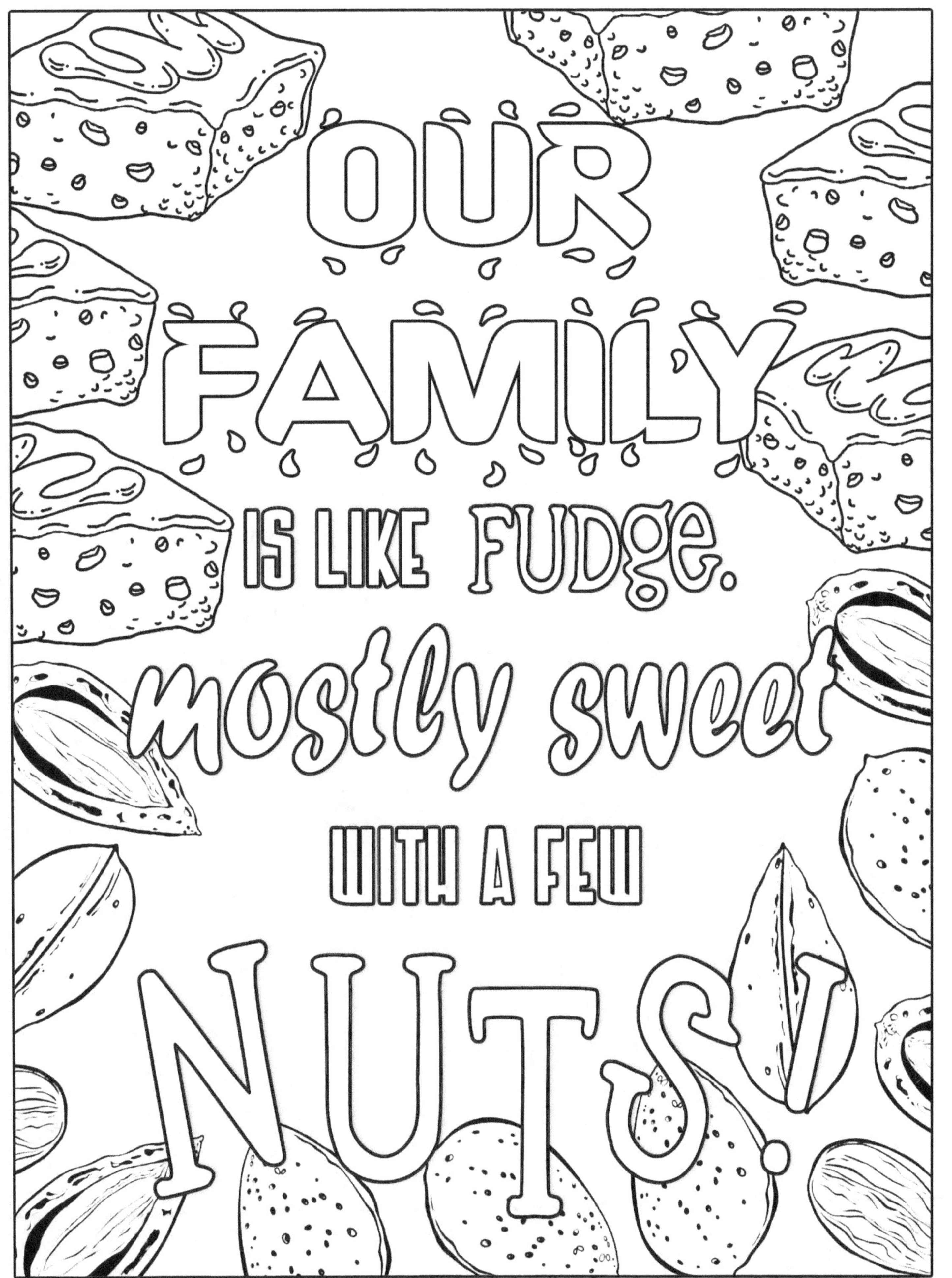

OUR
FAMILY
IS LIKE FUDGE.
mostly sweet
WITH A FEW
NUTS.

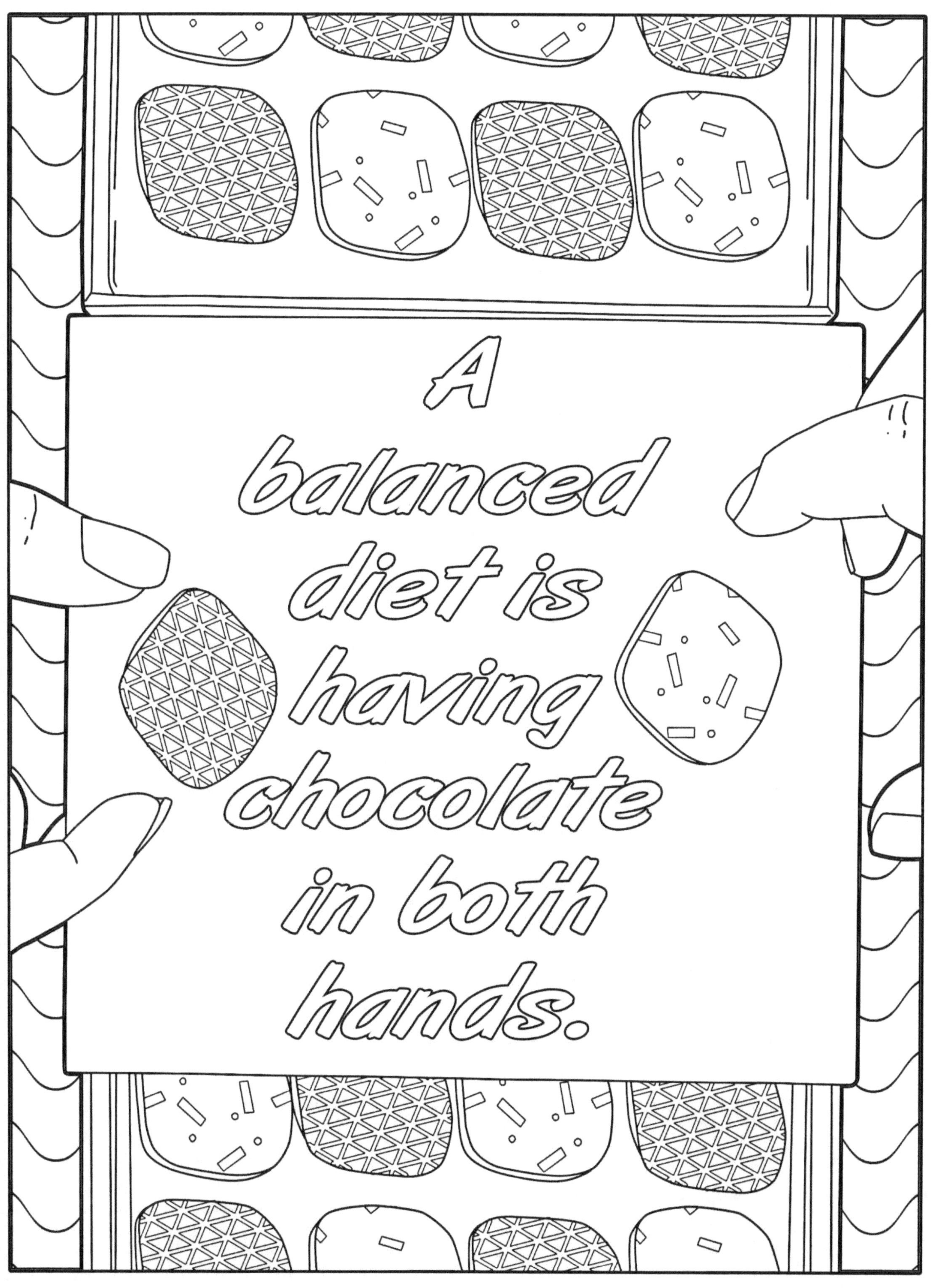

A
balanced
diet is
having
chocolate
in both
hands.

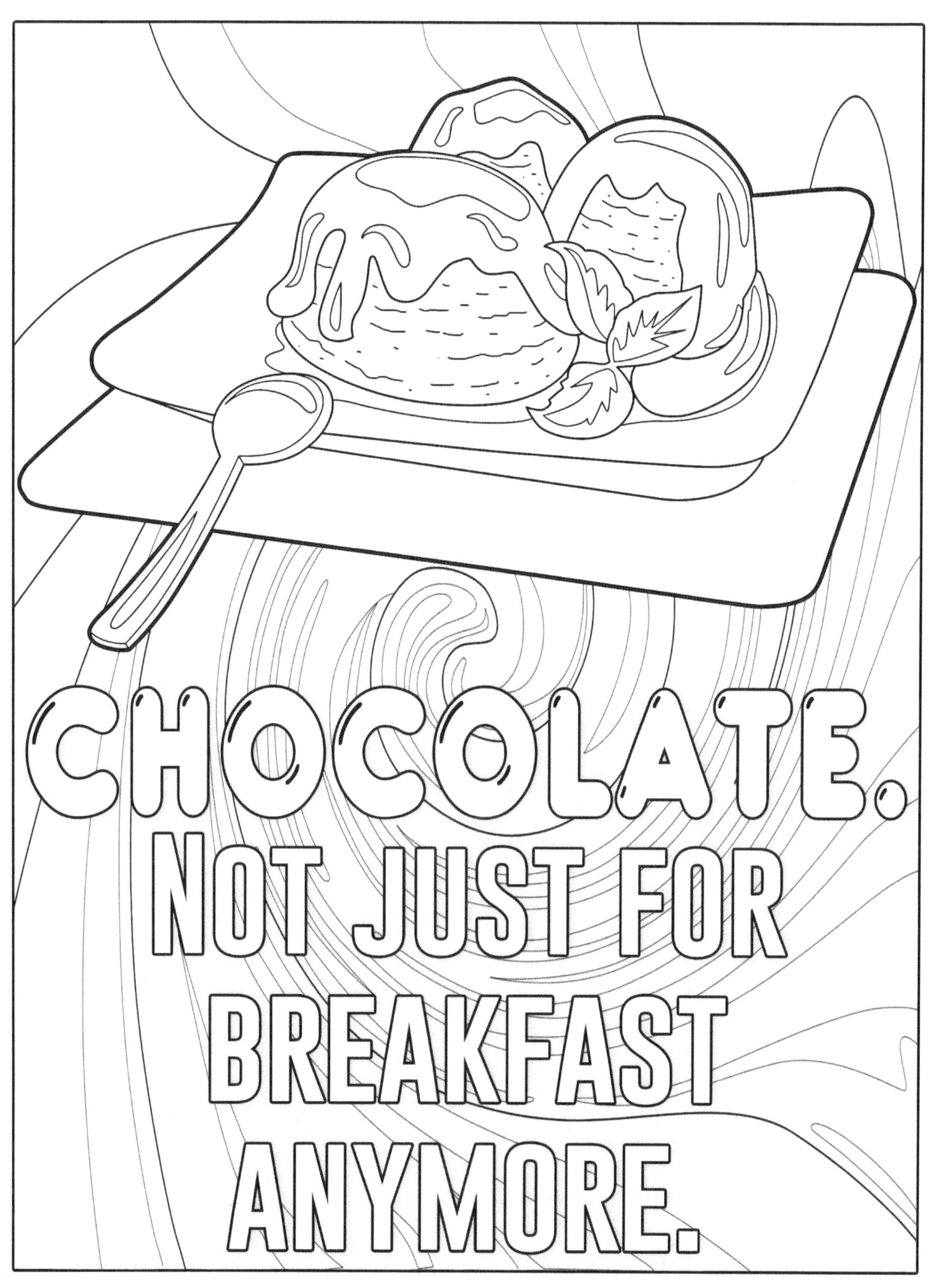

CHOCOLATE.
NOT JUST FOR
BREAKFAST
ANYMORE.

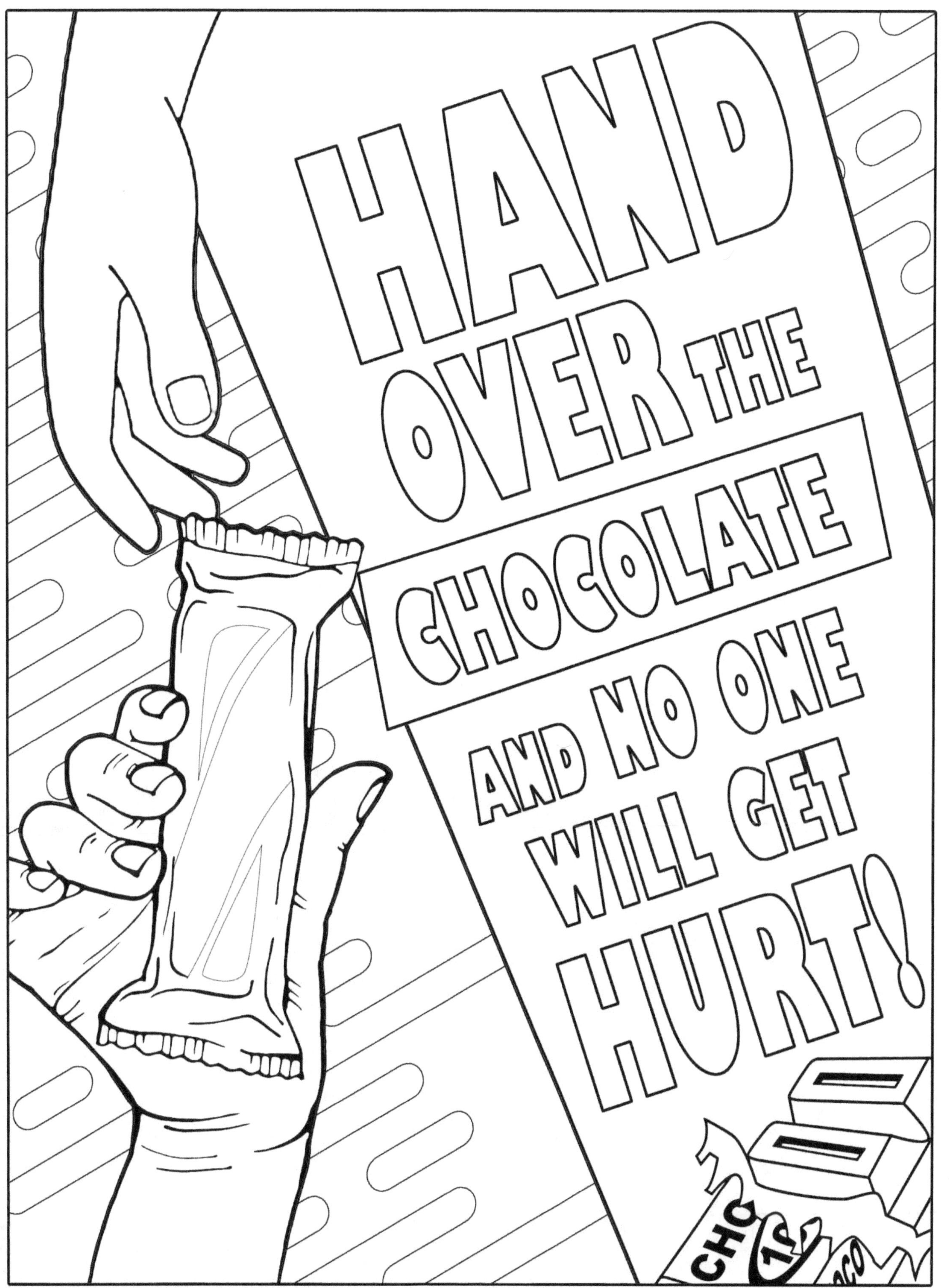

HAND
OVER THE
CHOCOLATE
AND NO ONE
WILL GET
HURT!

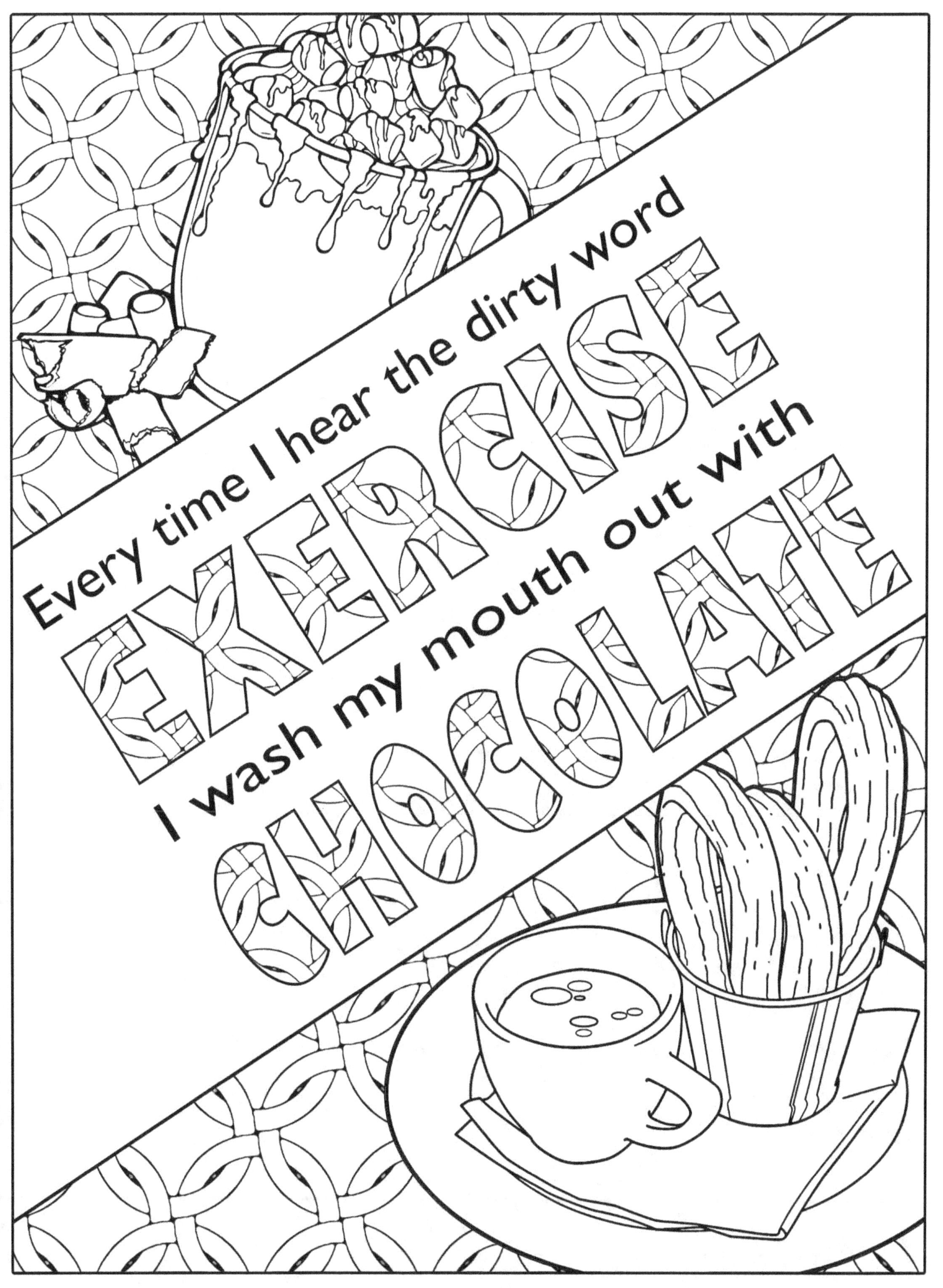
Every time I hear the dirty word
EXERCISE
I wash my mouth out with
CHOCOLATE

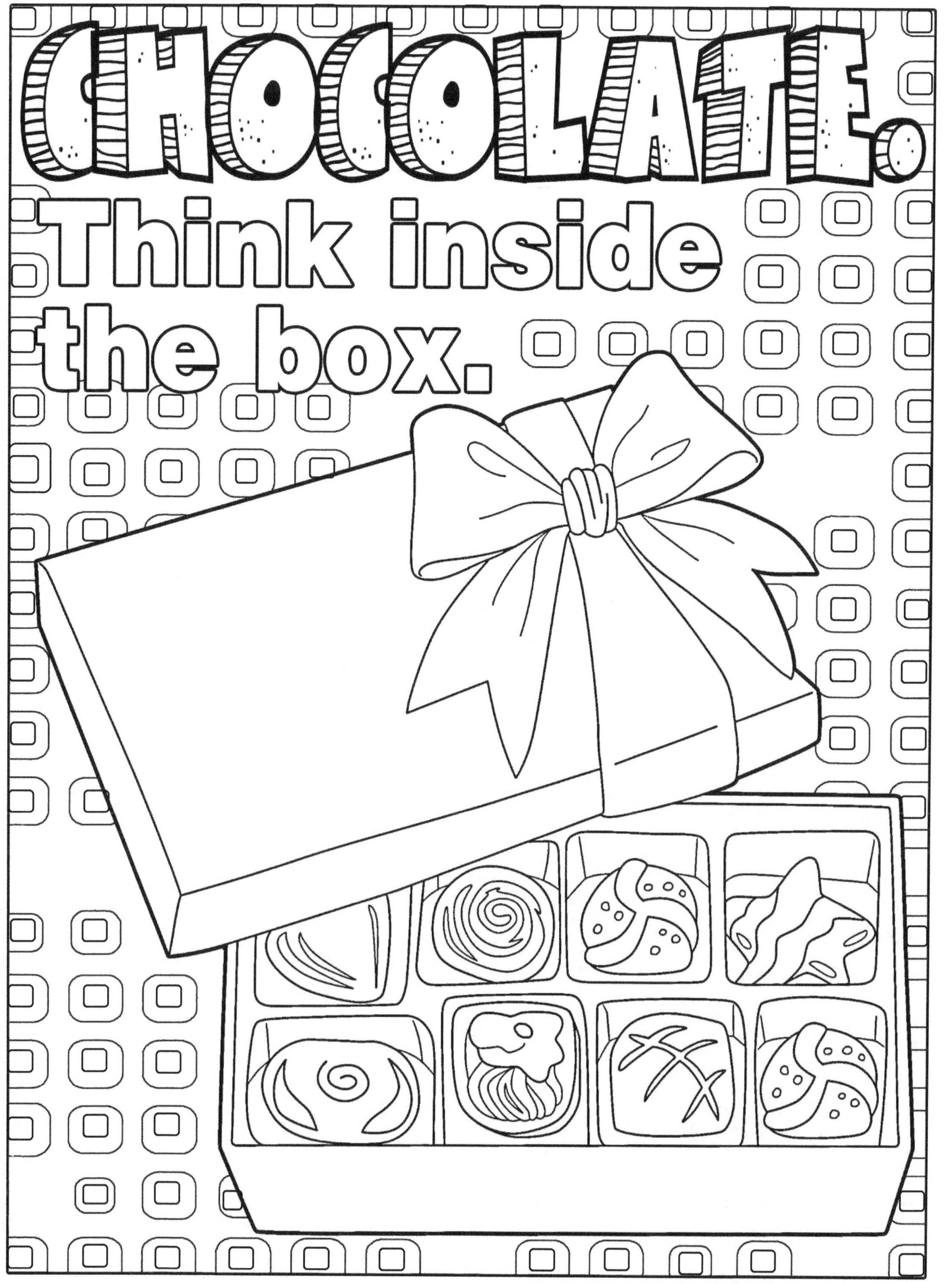

CHOCOLATE.
Think inside
the box.

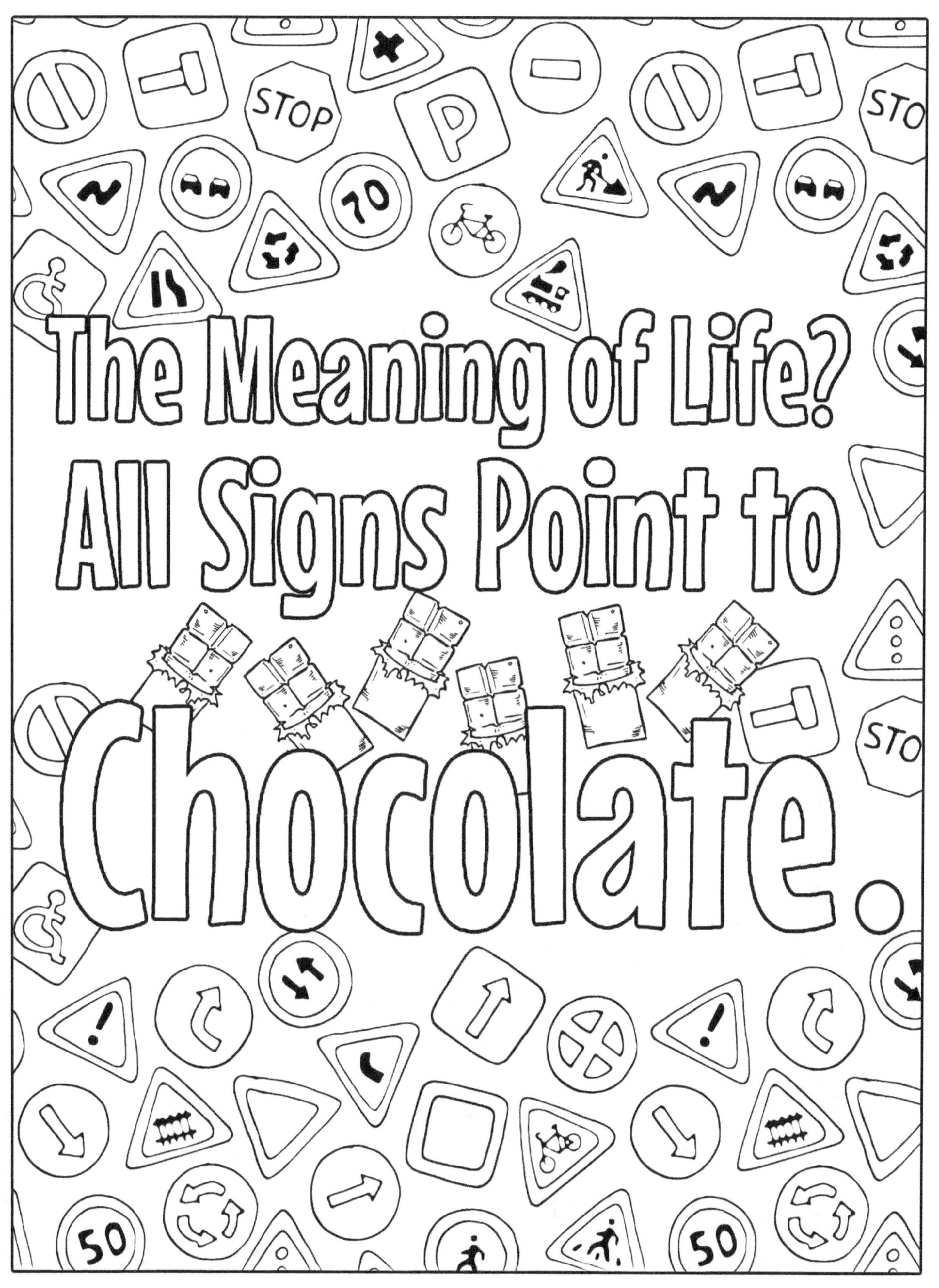

The Meaning of Life?
All Signs Point to
Chocolate.
STOP
STO
P
70
50
50

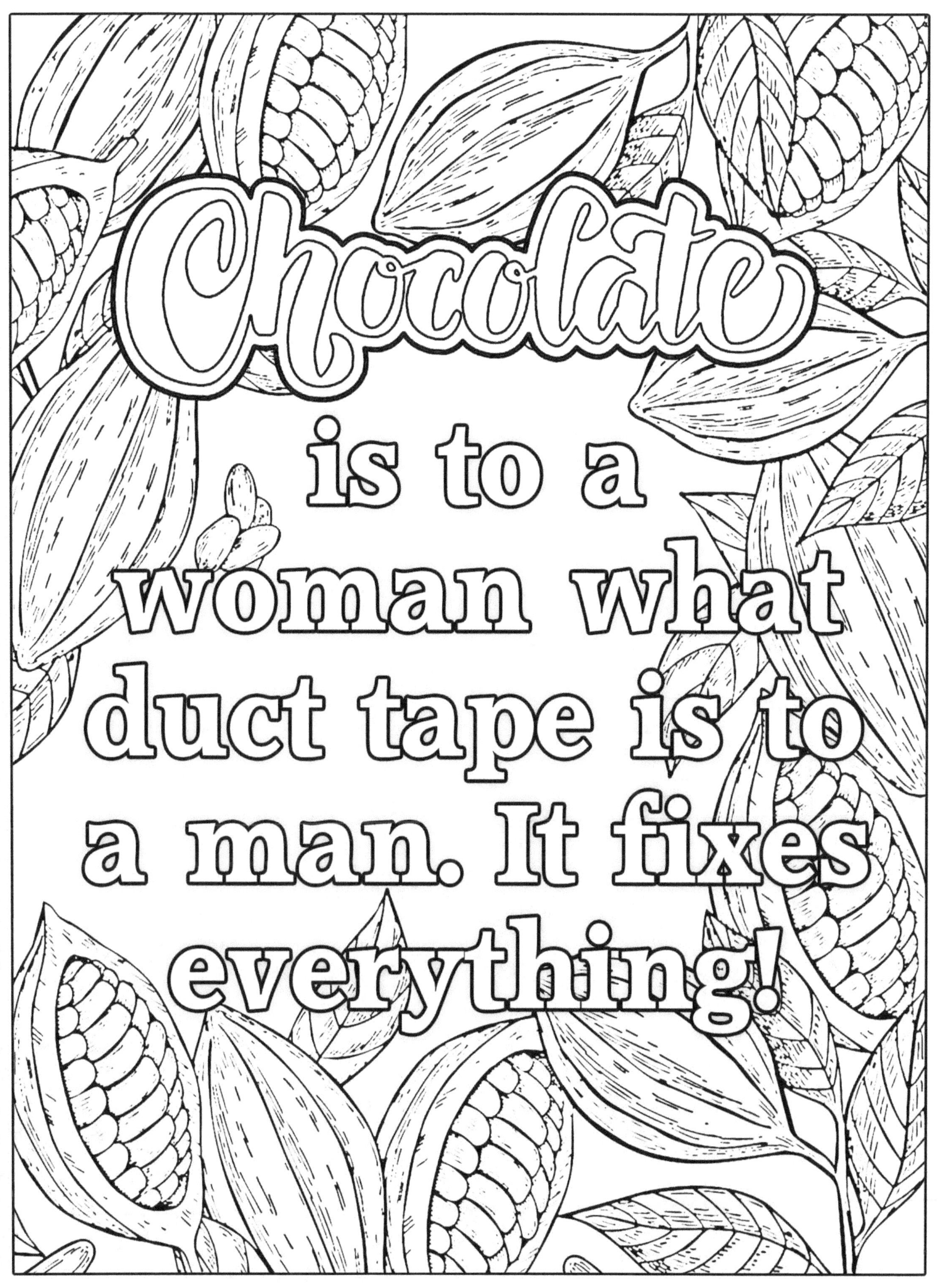

Chocolate
is to a woman what duct tape is to a man. It fixes everything!

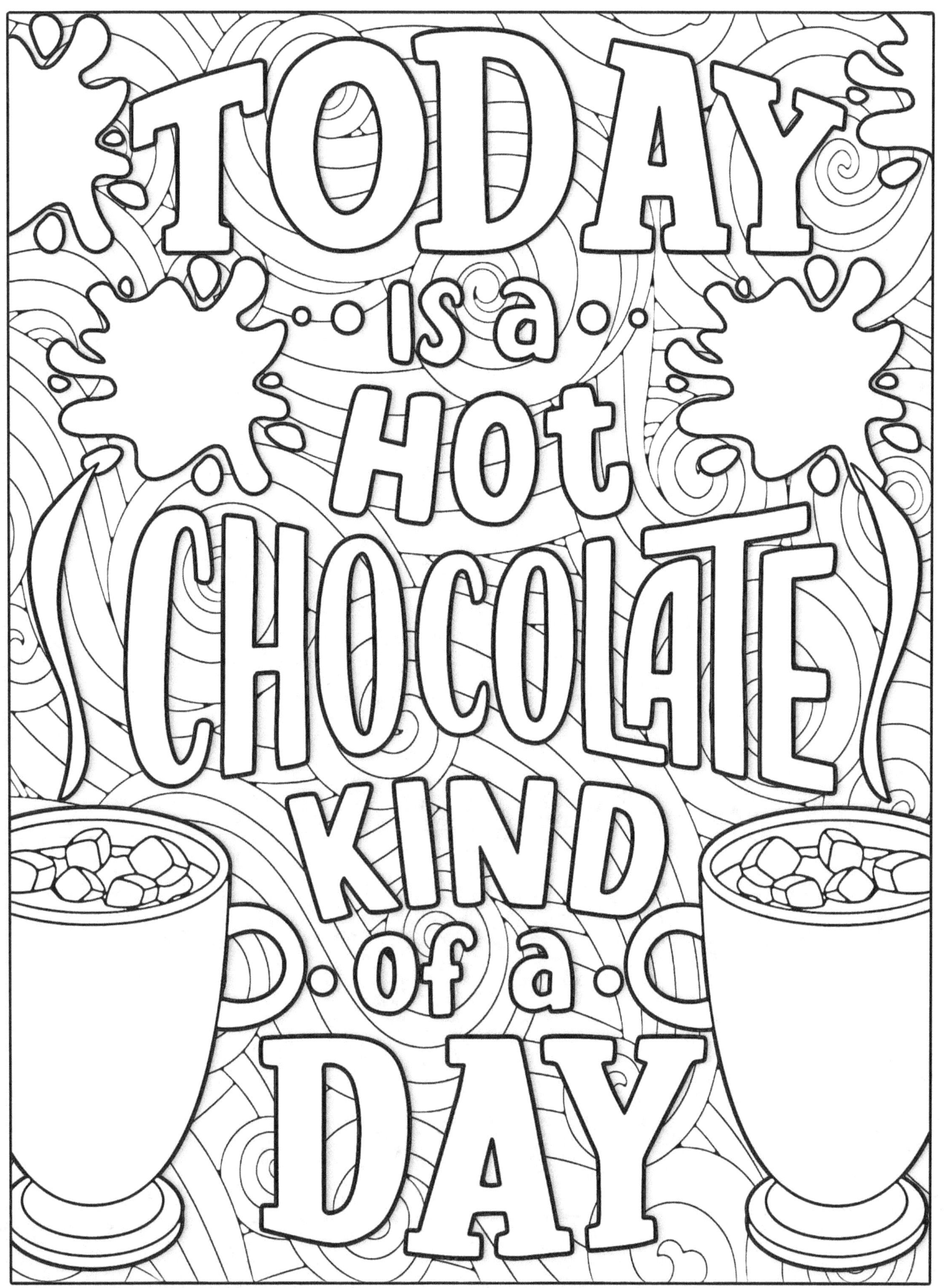

TODAY
is a
HOT
CHOCOLATE
KIND
of a
DAY

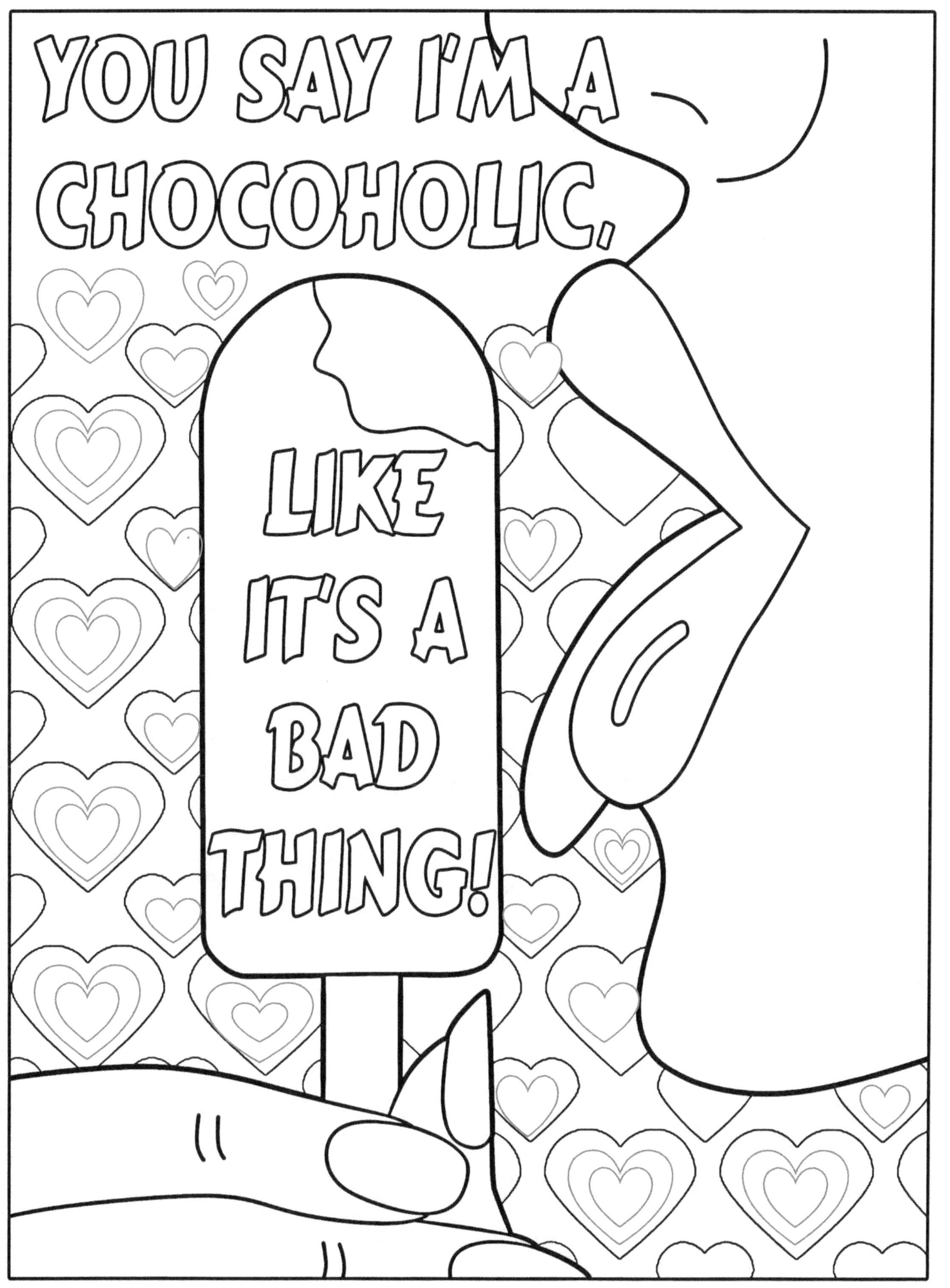

YOU SAY I'M A CHOCOHOLIC.
LIKE IT'S A BAD THING!

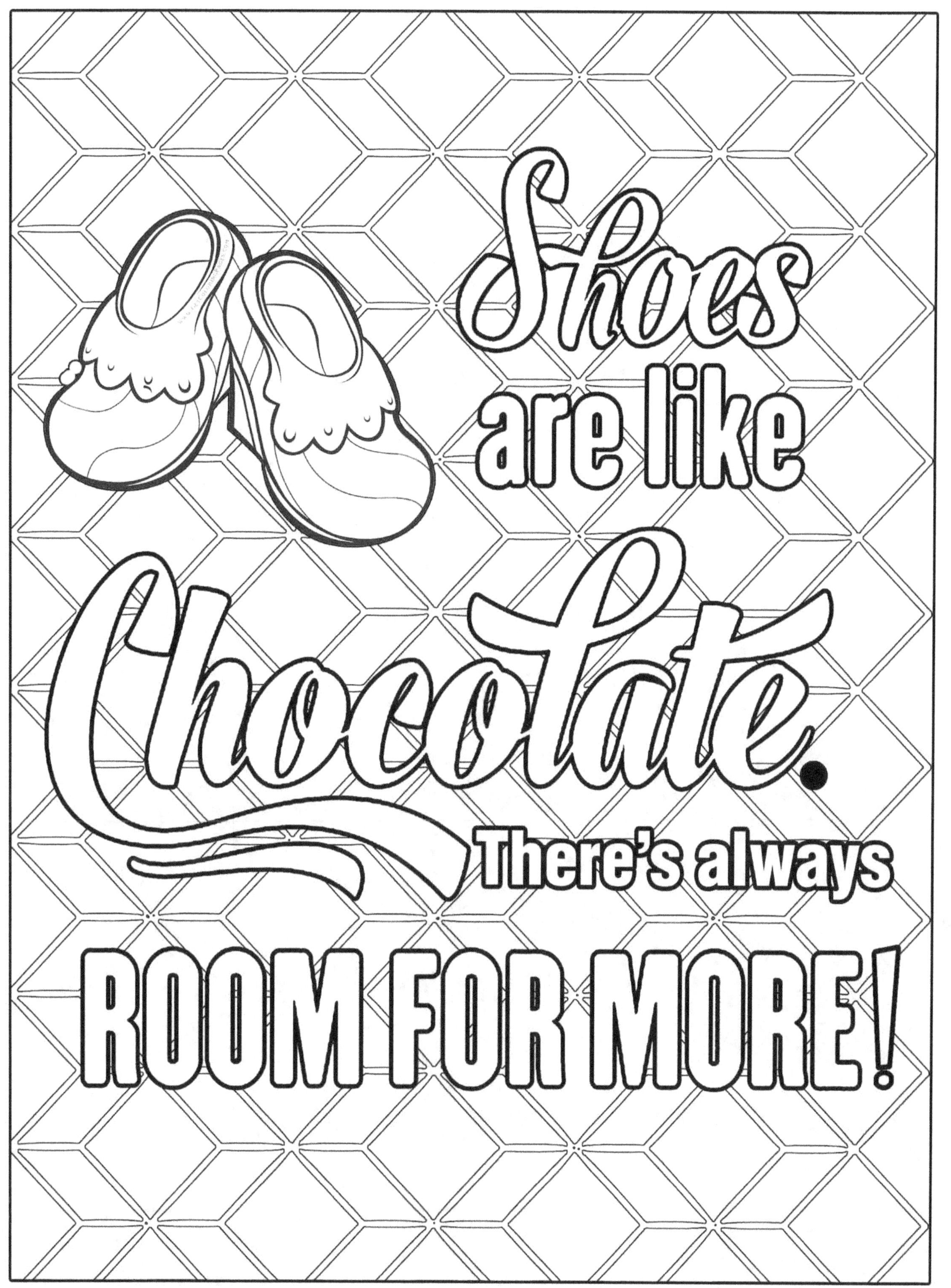

Shoes
are like
Chocolate.
There's always
ROOM FOR MORE!

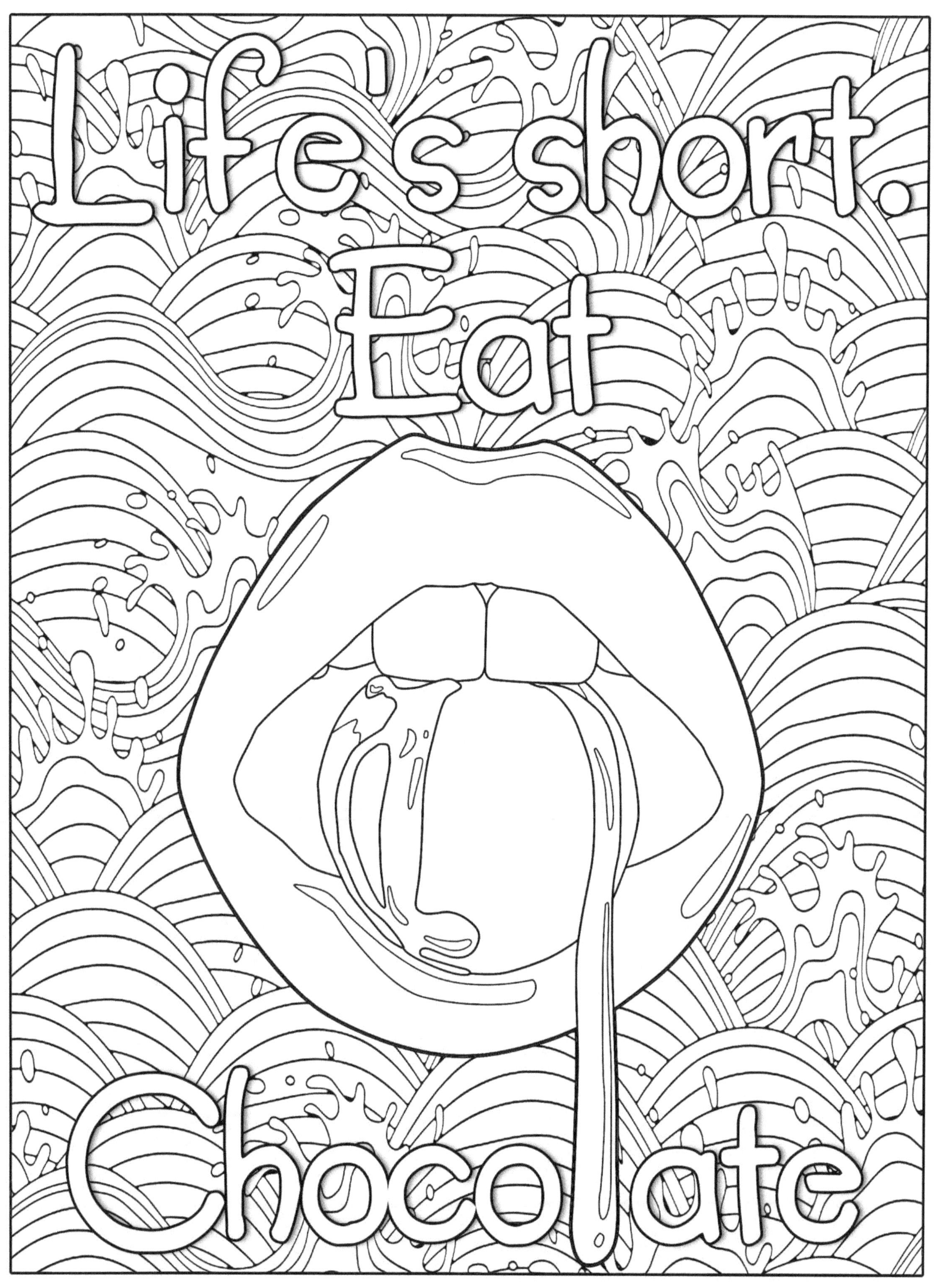

Life's short.
Eat
Chocolate

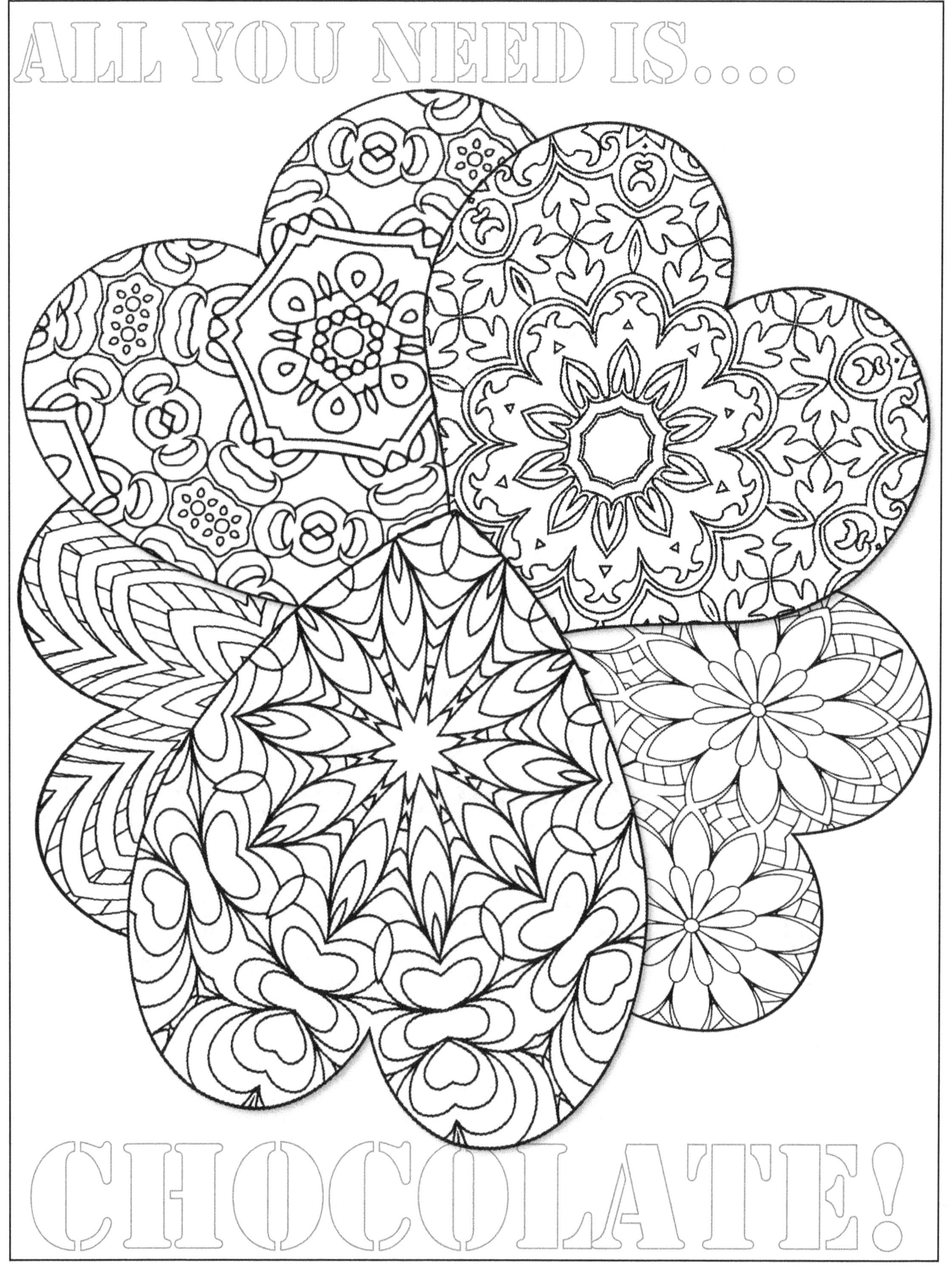

ALL YOU NEED IS....
CHOCOLATE!

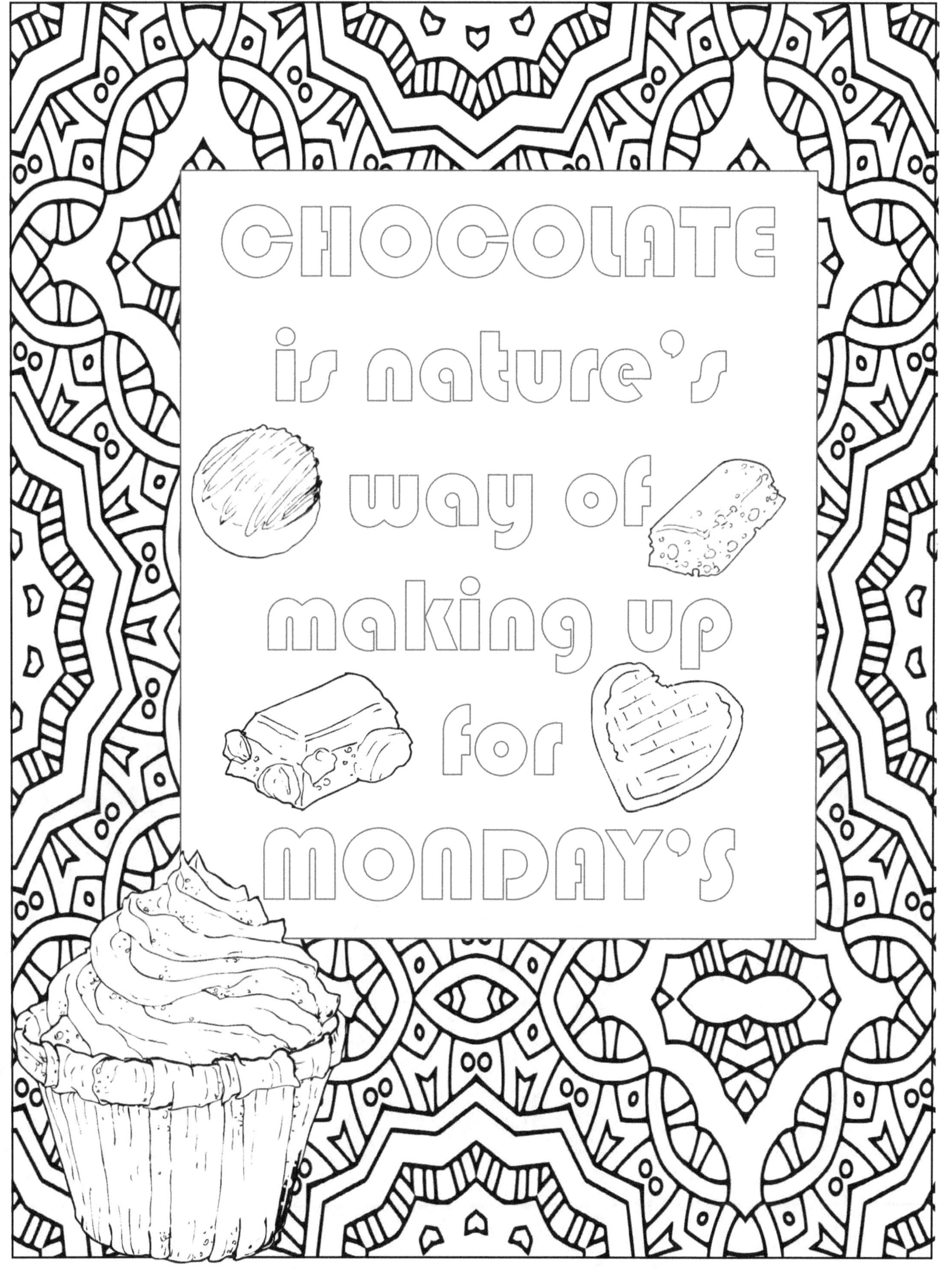

CHOCOLATE
is nature's
way of
making up
for
MONDAY'S

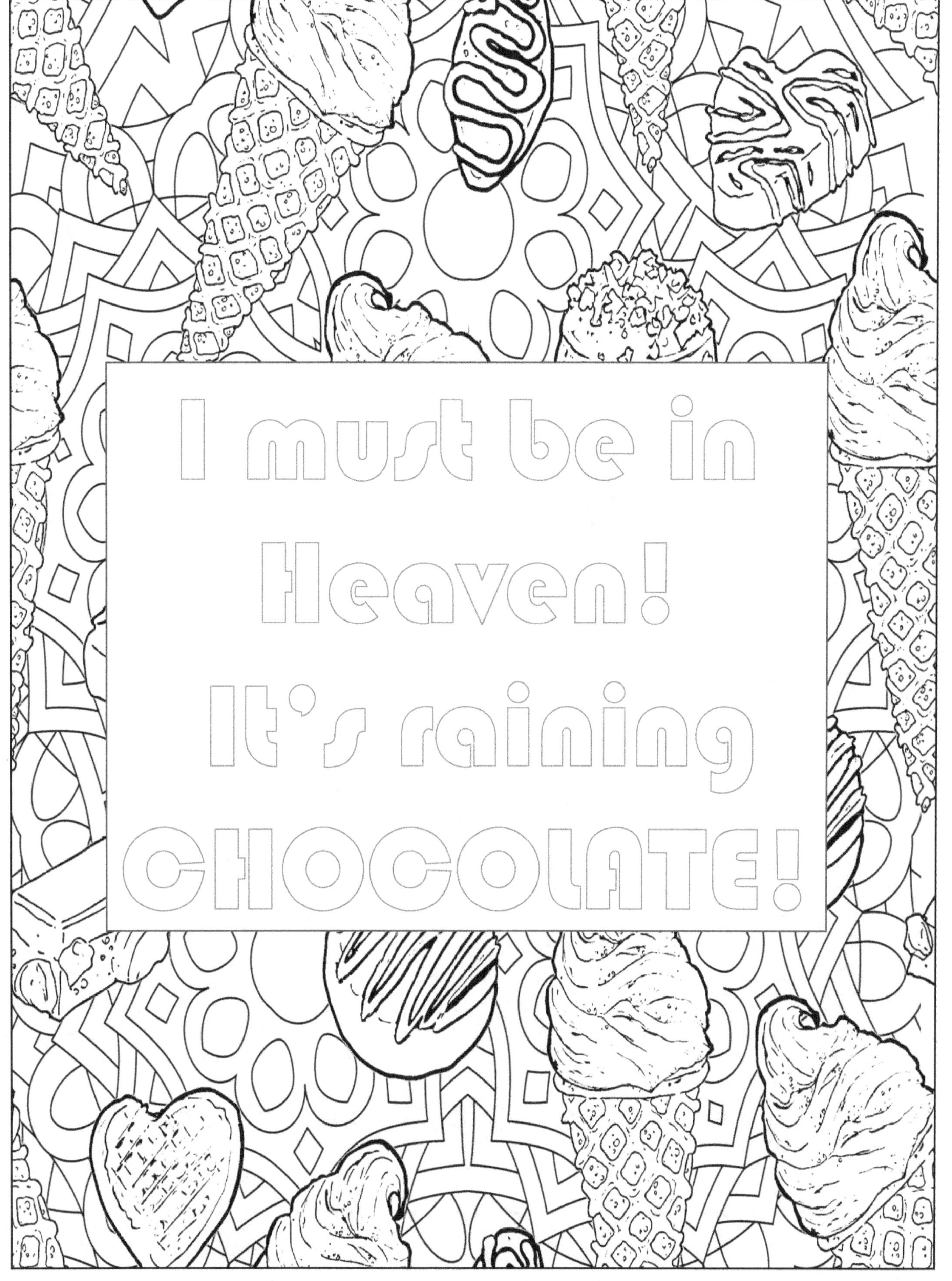

I must be in Heaven!
It's raining CHOCOLATE!

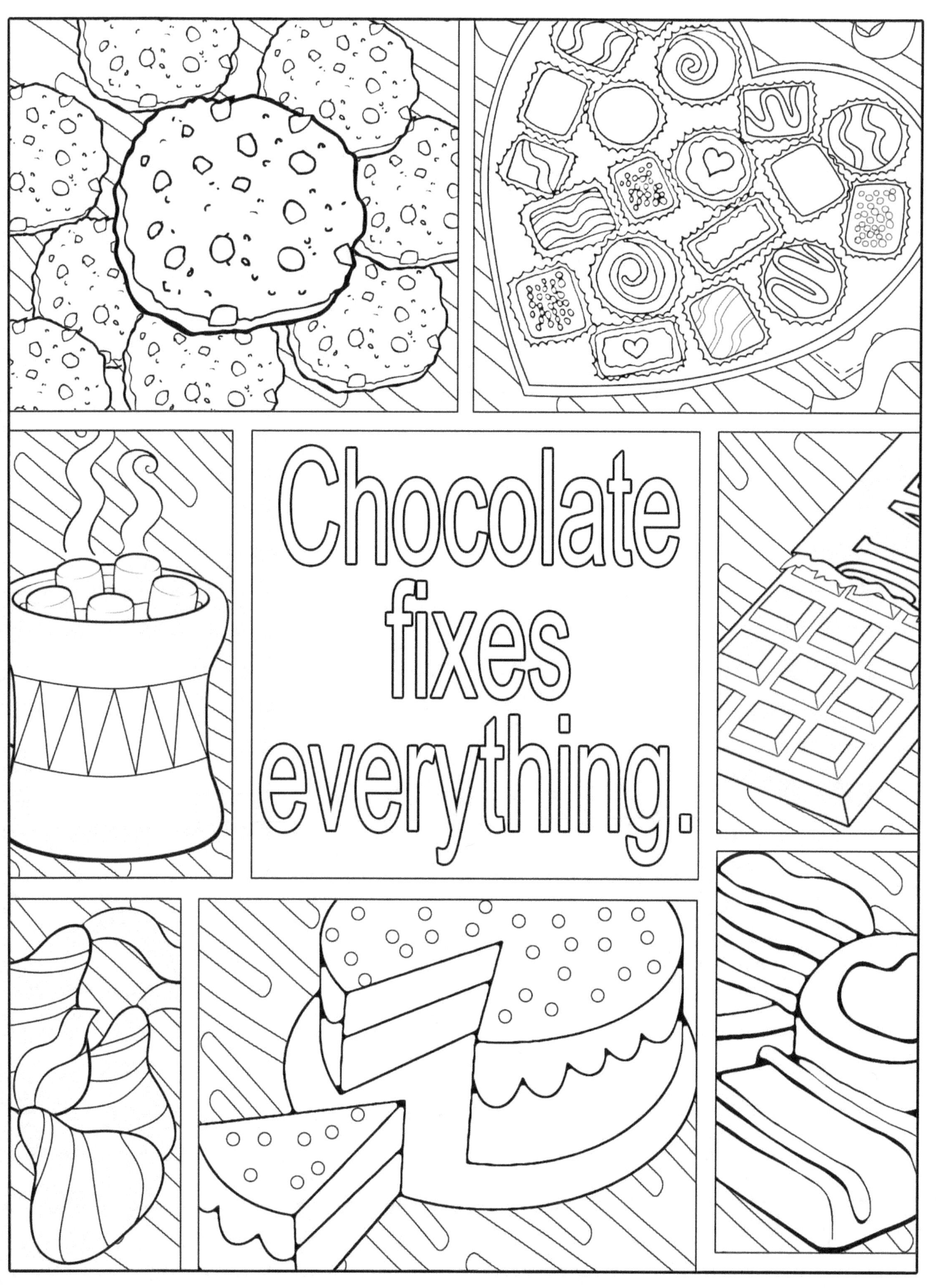
Chocolate
fixes
everything.

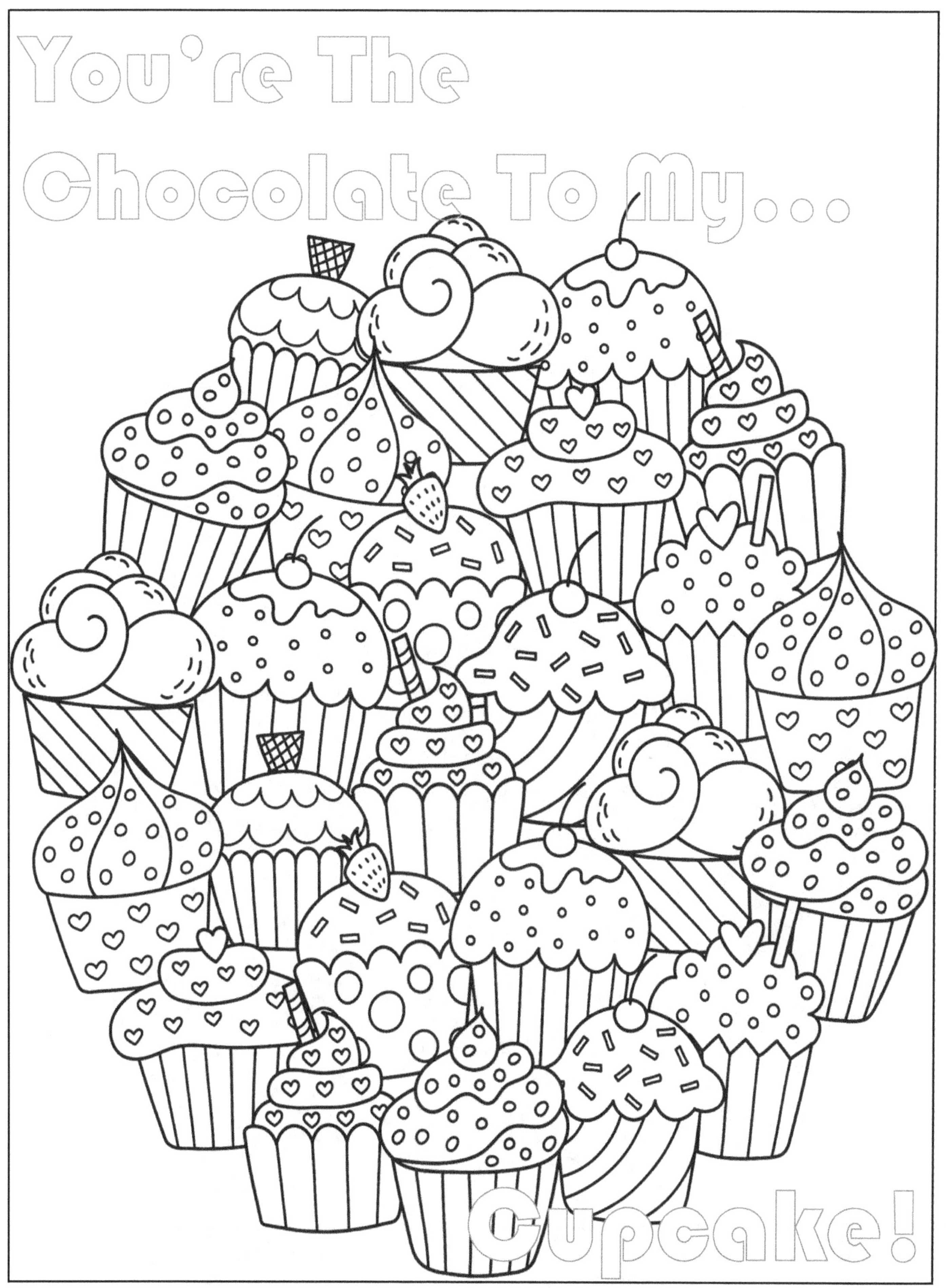

You're The
Chocolate To My...
Cupcake!

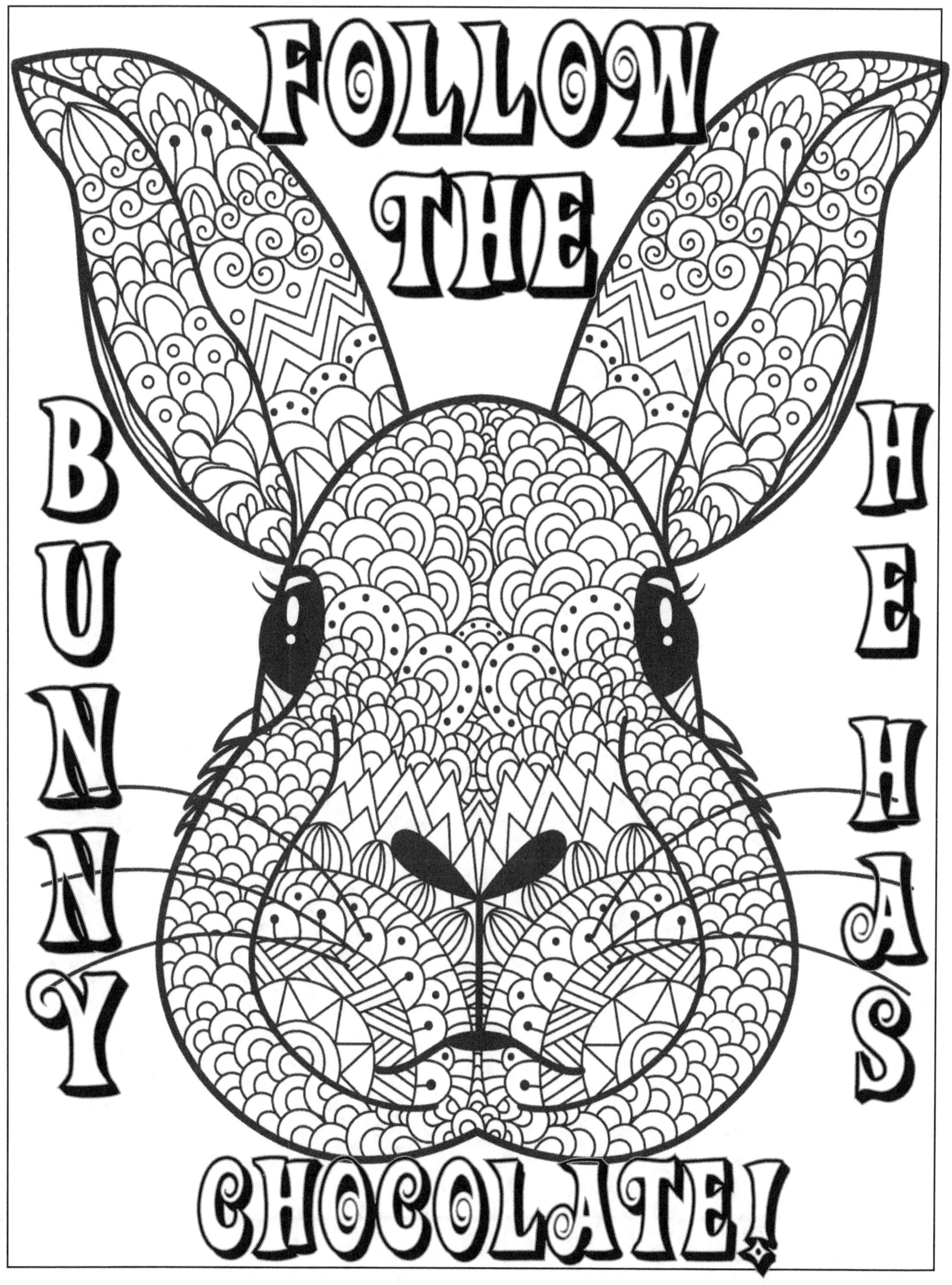

FOLLOW
THE
BUNNY
HE HAS
CHOCOLATE!

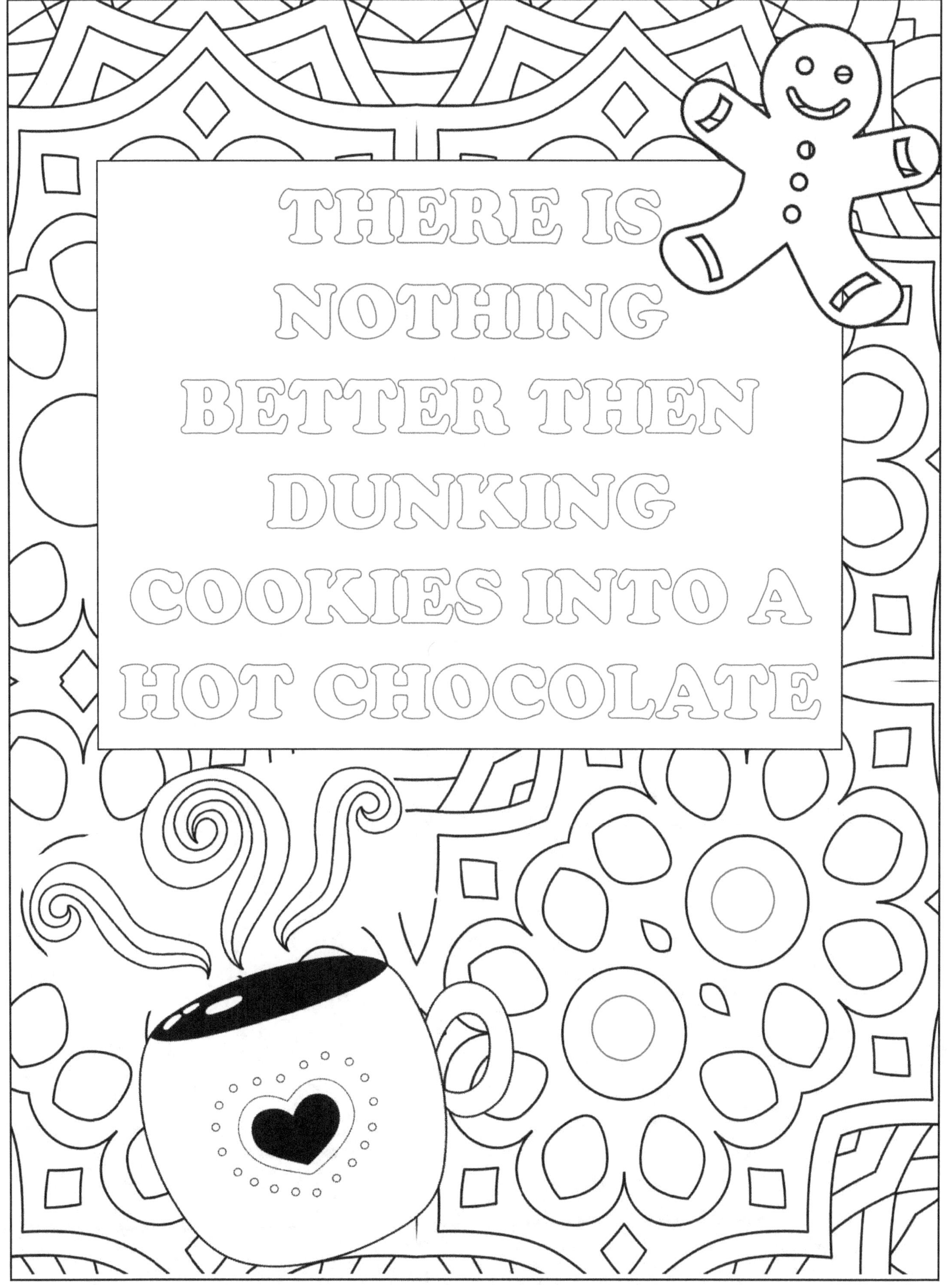

THERE IS NOTHING BETTER THEN DUNKING COOKIES INTO A HOT CHOCOLATE

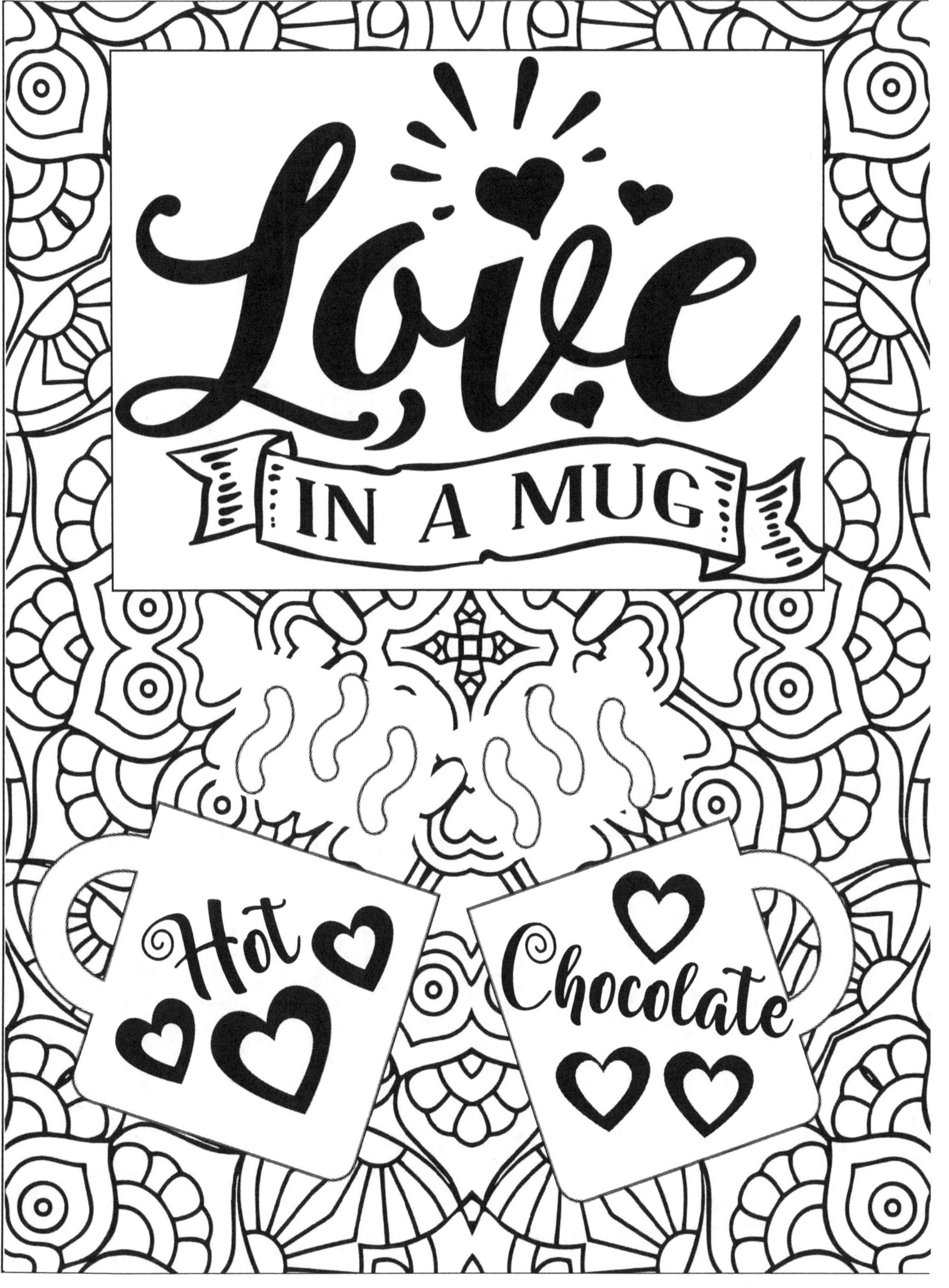

Love
IN A MUG
Hot
Chocolate

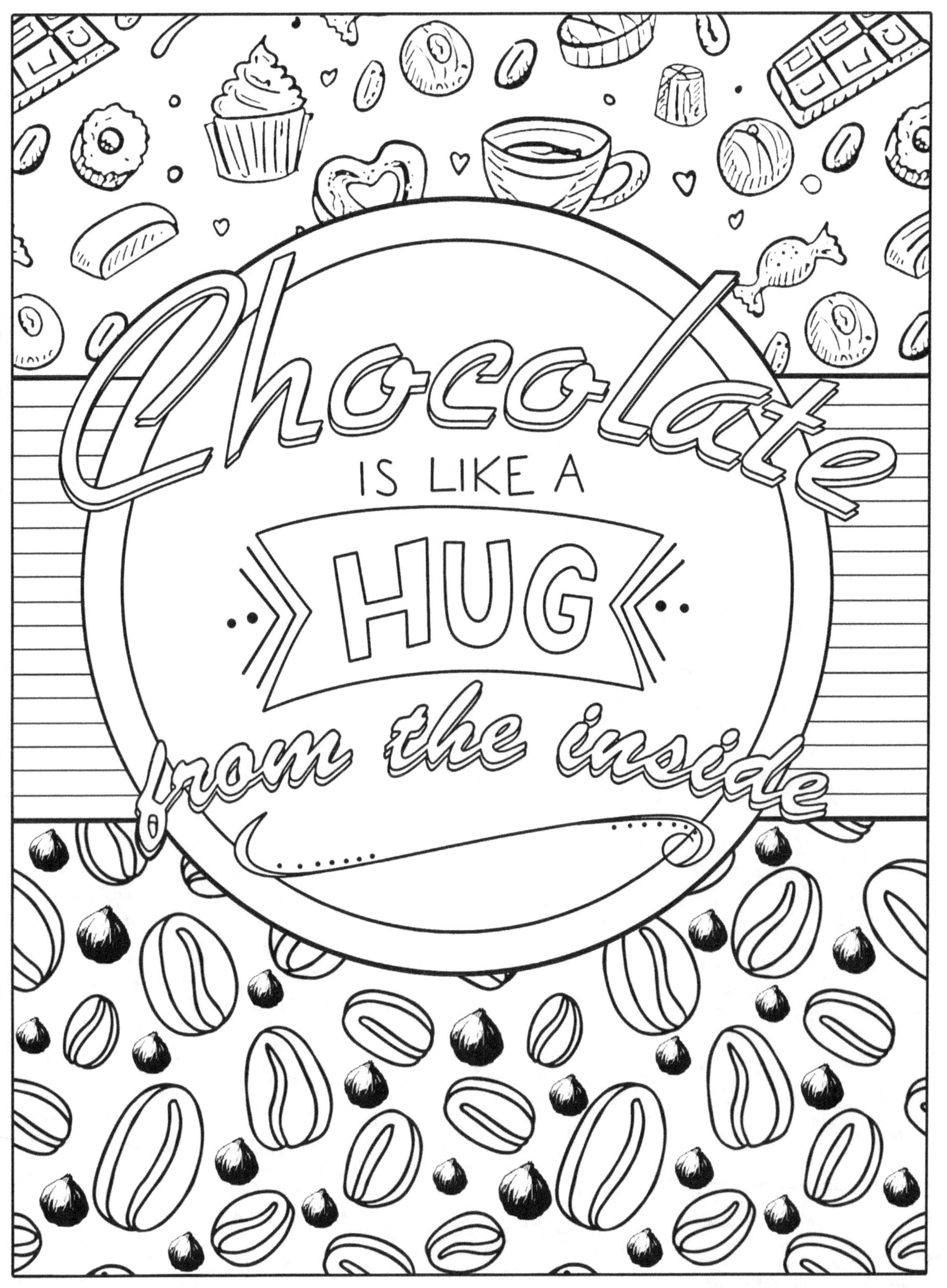

Chocolate
IS LIKE A
HUG
from the inside